Infertility and Identity

Lara L. Deveraux

Ann Jackoway Hammerman

10/00 Ann Hammerman

Infertility and Identity

New Strategies for Treatment

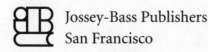

Jossey-Bass Publishers
San Francisco

Substantial discounts on bulk quantities of Jossey-Bass books are available to corporations, professional associations, and other organizations. For details and discount information, contact the special sales department at Jossey-Bass Inc., Publishers (415) 433–1740; Fax (800) 605–2665.

For sales outside the United States, please contact your local Simon & Schuster International Office.

www.josseybass.com

Manufactured in the United States of America on Lyons Falls Turin Book. This paper is acid-free and 100 percent totally chlorine-free.

Library of Congress Cataloging-in-Publication Data
Deveraux, Lara L., date.
   Infertility and identity : new strategies for treatment / Lara L.
Deveraux, Ann Jackoway Hammerman.
      p.   cm.
   Includes bibliographical references and index.
   ISBN 0-7879-3881-5
   1. Infertility—Treatment.   I. Hammerman, Ann Jackoway, date.
II. Title.
RC889.D483   1998
616.6'9206—dc21   97-49290

FIRST EDITION
HB Printing   10 9 8 7 6 5 4 3 2 1

⌒ Contents

    Appendix A: Suggested Viewing and Reading Lists   283

    Appendix B: Resources   288

    Appendix C: Alternatives to Biological Parenting   292

    References   305

    About the Authors   307

    Index   309

—⁀— Preface

Throughout this book we suggest that the condition of infertility can be incorporated into a client's identity, and we provide strategies for you to help them do that. To effectively apply our treatment model, please consider two things: one, that the cultural expectation to marry and have children (so often depicted in happily-ever-after tales) is but one possible road to happiness; and two, that the supposed biological *destiny* to procreate is, in actuality, a biological *possibility* to procreate. These two tenets of our therapeutic approach are what help us to assist clients on their journey to create lives they *can* live rather than lives they think they *should* be living.

It is a rare child of Western civilization who is not influenced by the profound cultural expectation to marry and have children. This expectation is incorporated into our identities and we grow up expecting these things from ourselves. So what happens if an individual never marries or never has children? How does he reconcile his lifestyle with the cultural expectations he has not manifested? We assert that he must redefine the path on which he will find happiness and fulfillment. This is particularly true for gay men and lesbians, and for individuals who remain single throughout their lives. For these clients we emphasize that the cultural expectations to marry and have children are merely options, not mandates. Clients who by our culture's standards are already living on the fringe of society through their choice of a same-sex partner or to have no partner at all are at risk of experiencing great despair if they pursue biological parenting and receive a diagnosis of infertility. This is because the inability to parent biologically is just one more element that denies the individual the opportunity to experience life in the cultural mainstream. But whether gay, single, or married, no one who receives a diagnosis of infertility is prepared to manage the implications of living this aspect of a life that is not defined by cultural standards.

And so they land at our doorsteps. We help clients who are experiencing infertility to shift from engaging in hot pursuit of a life they think they *should* be living, to defining a life they *can* live. We accept the awesome task of helping them to alleviate their despair over not manifesting the traditionally accepted path to happily ever after. By helping our clients to accept and incorporate infertility into their identities, they become able to create their own definitions of happiness.

In this politically correct era, when allowable reactions to the entire gamut of lifestyles range from tolerance (at the very least) to celebration (at the very most), there lies another perspective: acceptance. Our present-day attitude toward the variety of ethnicities, religions, and lifestyle choices that make up our world espouses acceptance of others and acceptance of ourselves. It is in the light of accepting infertility that we have written this book. This book is our stand against the pressure clients feel to make their lives conform to societal norms, and it is our stand in favor of helping these clients make conscious, responsible choices for living whole, fulfilled lives.

ACKNOWLEDGMENTS

We gratefully acknowledge all of the writers from whom we have quoted for their inspiration. We also thank the following individuals for their invaluable contributions to our efforts: Kathleen Scogna, David Brake, Joanne Clapp Fullagar, Michele Jones, Barbara Hill, Katie Levine, Cinderella, Karen Sharpe, Alan Rinzler, Dr. Robert Nachtigall, Jean Caine, Rosette Gossett-Signorelli, Teri Clemens, Linda Perilstein, Dr. Sherman Silber and his support staff, Dudley Dunlop, RESOLVE, and our clients.

Ann extends her gratitude to Jeff and Leslie Newcorn, Landmark, Catherine McHugh, Mike and Judy Newmark, Greg and Aida Parnas, Emily Sutterfield, Congregation Neve Shalom, Ray Chance, Linda Bridges, Diana Randall, Maureen Ellis, Yvonne Jackson, Pat and Geta Jackoway, Maryann Mica, Marc and Nancy Hammerman, Jon Jackoway and Alan Peabody, and Emily, Jordan, and Doug Hammerman.

Lara thanks her sisters, Kristi, Tana, Kat, Moe, Beth, and Lori. She also thanks Brad Hines, Craig Swett, Cynthia Webster, Teri McCarthy, Paulette Foerster, Jayme, Matthew, and Jacob Dawson, and Adam and Ryan Swett.

St. Louis, Missouri   LARA L. DEVERAUX
March 1998   ANN JACKOWAY HAMMERMAN

Infertility and Identity

This book is dedicated to my parents

Phyllis and Harris Jackoway

—AJH

For my parents

Beth and Arlyn

—LLD

Introduction

Freedom is the will to be responsible to ourselves.

—*Nietzsche*, Twilight of the Idols

During our combined twenty years of clinical experience we have consistently struggled to find and develop treatment strategies for our clients who have been diagnosed with infertility. When we began working with clients who were experiencing infertility, we could offer them little more than the basic counseling skills we had learned during our college and graduate schooling. At the time we were both employed as adoption facilitators, and most of our clients came to us three to six years after they had received their initial infertility diagnosis. It was striking to us that when we asked our prospective adoptive parents about their experience with infertility, we would almost always hear one of two very dissimilar responses: our clients would either start to cry and subsequently apologize for their reaction, or they would offer a seemingly detached and clinical explanation of their experiences.

Because we had been instructed to determine whether or not our clients had resolved their infertility, their reactions confused us: neither of these reactions seemed to indicate a state of resolution. We were also at a loss to understand why there seemed to be such an absence of a middle ground in their reactions. As we began to educate ourselves about infertility, through reading and discussions with our clients and each other, we also began to recognize the connections between infertility, grief, and loss. Once we were able to make a clear connection between grief and infertility we realized that we had been looking for *resolution* of the infertility—an event—when we should have been looking for stages of acceptance—a process.

It was at this point that we began to understand our clients' reactions to our questions about their experience with infertility. If they too were looking for resolution, and like us were unable to blend the infertility experience with the concept of resolution, it was not surprising that their reactions were extreme. Not surprising because our clients were fully aware that resolution was generally thought to be the healthiest outcome of an experience with infertility. And as *resolution of grief* is an oxymoron, the emphasis placed on resolution was leading to repression of our clients' emotions. And repression of emotions often results in fluctuations between emotional detachment and rushes of intense emotion.

Although we found traditional models of grief therapy to be helpful in our pursuit of understanding our clients' reactions to infertility, we also found them lacking in their ability to fully address infertility. Our experience with our clients has shown us that infertility not only elicits a grief reaction but also assaults our clients' most basic assumptions about their bodies, their potential roles as parents, and their ideas about what it means to be male or female, and shatters their cultural and innate assumptions about their right and ability to procreate. In short, traditional grief therapy models simply did not address the impact that infertility seemed to be having on our clients' identities.

Not only did traditional models of grief therapy fail to address the relationship between infertility and identity, but none of the resources that dealt with infertility provided any information either. This lack of information on the psychosocial aspects of infertility further complicated our attempts to develop treatment strategies for our clients. Although we knew that mental health professionals would be the most likely population to research and develop psychosocial treatment strategies for infertility, we found that ethical, knowledge-based treatment strategies for infertility were almost nonexistent. The psychosocial symptoms associated with an infertility diagnosis may persist during or after a pregnancy or an adoption; without practice-based research to support that ongoing psychological distress common among clients experiencing infertility, therapists are at risk for viewing this distress as pathological.

Infertility issues are not formally taught in schools of social work or other training programs for mental health professionals or therapists and are not, therefore, usually considered as worthy of further investigation. The lack of formal training is surprising indeed, when you consider that in the United States alone infertility currently affects approximately 4.9 million people. Infertility is also overlooked by the mental health industry.

Infertility is not even addressed in the *DSM-IV,* although other matters of reproduction are (such as PMS and issues related to pregnancy). When mental health professionals *do* address infertility, they most often do so *after* an individual has experienced problems with fertility.

Meanwhile, however, developments in reproductive technology are at an all-time high. In addition, bookstore shelves are lined with personal accounts of authors' infertility experiences, with self-help manuals by pseudo-professionals, and with dozens of books that teach consumers how to adopt children.

AUDIENCE

This book is significantly different from others on the market because it is written for therapists and offers them new strategies for treating clients who are experiencing infertility. Our approach has been to seek a path that leads clients to an integration of the losses of infertility into their identities, to a regained sense of wholeness. The book is designed to provide you with an understanding of the unique issues associated with infertility; tools to assess those issues in relationships; and treatment guidelines for therapists working with clients who are experiencing this widely ignored life crisis.

This book also explains the tasks required for *acceptance* of infertility. Facilitating acceptance of infertility is one of our key themes because much of the current literature and research focuses on the medical aspects of infertility and on the various reproductive technologies that are available to overcome it. We have chosen to focus on the aspects of infertility that our clients most often manifest: grief, and difficulties integrating the infertility into their identities. Acceptance of infertility is the outcome of a therapeutic process that facilitates the grief process and the integration of infertility into identity.

It is important to note that this book is an essential part of the education of any professional who is involved in adoption or in counseling clients who have been affected by adoption. Research and our experience support the premise that adopted individuals are overrepresented in the population seeking help from social workers, psychologists, and psychiatrists. Because an exceptionally high percentage of couples diagnosed with infertility who are subsequently unable to have biological children eventually become adoptive parents, it is imperative that all mental health professionals understand the context within which many adoptions take place: a context of loss. Adoptees often internalize their adoptive parents' loss of a biological child, and they subsequently seek counseling in an attempt to resolve the legacy of that loss. Therefore, in addition to counseling couples with infertility, mental health professionals must be prepared to counsel adopted children, adult adoptees, biological families of adopted children (biological families most often seek counseling after their biological child has contacted them), or adoptive parents.

This book is also appropriate for members of the clergy, because they are in a position to educate and support the members of their congregations who are experiencing infertility. Other professionals that clients will encounter when they are experiencing fertility problems, such as physicians, attorneys, and adoption facilitators can also benefit from this book. Although each of these professionals will deal with different aspects of infertility—for example, by providing medical intervention or advice on the legal aspects of alternatives to biological parenting, or by facilitating an adoption—they all must be aware of the unique impact of infertility on the client.

In this era of managed health care, when mental health benefits are limited in scope and duration, we would be remiss if we presented practitioners with treatment strategies that were not applicable to their managed care clients. Our treatment plan meets the criteria for managed care companies because it offers clearly structured, solution-focused, and time-limited plans for intervention. We also provide "managed care–friendly" and sequential session plans; comprehensive explanations of typical client responses to an infertility diagnosis, failed treatment, and pregnancy loss; and a discussion on the alternatives to biological parenting, which include the options to remain child-free or to pursue parenting through adoption.

Because our clients come to us when they are in the initial stages of medical treatment, or after their children have grown up and left home, and everywhere in between, we have designed our treatment approach to be applicable at any stage in our clients' experience with infertility. Although the issues that clients present vary with their stage of life, we have learned that integration of the infertility experience into our clients' identities is a task that must be reaccomplished throughout the life cycle. Therefore, the information and case examples we provide demonstrate the application of our approach throughout the life cycle.

OVERVIEW OF THE CONTENTS

This book is organized into four parts. Part One, "Preparing the Therapist," explains our new model of treatment; equips you with an understanding of the therapeutic skills that we have found to be most effective with our clients; and identifies the repercussions of an infertility diagnosis and specifically addresses the loss of normal functioning and the impact that gender has on our clients' reactions to infertility.

Part Two, "Understanding the Client Experience with Infertility," presents therapists with the perspective of infertility as a life crisis. We explore the influence that culture has on how our clients respond to reproductive losses (losses such as miscarriage, the loss of the potential biological child, and the loss of reproductive autonomy). We also examine the profound impact infertility has on sexuality.

Part Three, "Strategies for Treatment," offers strategies for facilitating the integration of infertility into the client's core identity and demonstrates why the task of integration must be reaccomplished throughout the life cycle. We also provide a thorough overview of the emotional implications of each available alternative to biological parenting.

Part Four, "Practical Applications," provides you with twelve session samples that offer guidance, session objectives, case examples, exercises that can be used in or outside the sessions, and strategies for the application of our theories, in order to assist you in developing a treatment plan for your clients.

The book also includes three appendixes. Appendix A consists of lists of movies and fiction and nonfiction books that we have found useful in our work with our clients and that are representative of our model of treatment in contexts that are not infertility specific. We recommend these titles to our clients in the hope that they will see that our approach to infertility counseling can be applied to other areas of their life and relationships. Appendix B is a list of resources for support groups, information on medical technology, information on alternatives to biological parenting, and newsletters that address specific client concerns. Appendix C outlines the practical considerations related to the various alternatives to biological parenting.

Throughout this book we emphasize the following key themes:

- Integrating infertility into identity
- Empowering clients
- Managing infertility in a fertility-focused world
- Challenging the myth that the best helpers are those who have experienced infertility
- Seeing loss and grief as inherent aspects of infertility

The following tools provide you with tangible applications of our approach:

- An explanation of therapeutic skills as they apply to infertility counseling
- Case examples
- Exercises for the client during each stage of the therapeutic process
- Homework assignments
- Reading and viewing lists that examine the indisputable connections between our challenges, our choices, and our fate
- A list of resources that can provide you and your clients with support, education, and additional resources

In summary, this book challenges the misleading assumption that pregnancy or adoption are "cures" for infertility. In fact, we challenge the notion that a successful outcome of infertility treatment and counseling must include parenthood or psychological resolution of the infertility. In support of this belief, we discuss the little-considered option of child-free living as a viable alternative, one that views parenting, reproduction, and parenthood as choices rather than as essential components of the happily-ever-after myth; we also discuss the need for therapists and clients to acknowledge that infertility forever changes a person's approach to marriage, parenthood, and his or her negotiation of the remaining stages of life.

We believe that our job as therapists is to guide our clients through the challenges that life presents, strengthen their sense of who they are, and help them see that they have the power to determine whether their experiences will shape them or destroy them. We have incorporated our clients' stories, their coping skills, their wisdom, and their strategies for effectively managing their infertility into our philosophy of treatment. We hope that our model will help you empower your clients to make choices that will facilitate the integration of their experience with infertility into their identities and subsequently enrich their lives.

We know that what we have to say is different from what others are currently saying. We may raise a few eyebrows and ruffle a few feathers. But our clients have taught us that these strategies work. It's time for a new approach.

PART ONE

Preparing the Therapist

*If your mind is empty, it is always ready for anything;
it is open to everything. In the beginner's mind there
are many possibilities, but in the expert's there are few.
—Shunryu Suzuki*

P art One includes Chapter One, "Pioneering a New Model of
Treatment," and Chapter Two, "Learning the Essential Skills of
Infertility Counseling." These two chapters are designed to educate you about our approach to infertility counseling and to present
the theoretical framework that is integral to the application of our
treatment approach. Chapter One explains why and how our model
of treatment emphasizes infertility as a condition, encourages clients
to acknowledge their losses, fosters client empowerment, and recog-
nizes and treats the impact of special concerns. Chapter Two identifies communication and guiding skills and explains why these skills
are essential to infertility counseling.

Pioneering a New Model of Treatment

Healing is used in the context of repair and restoration, integration, and wholeness. Healing is not necessarily curing. Healing is softening, opening, integrating, reaching for the depths of our feelings.

—Rabbi James Stone Goodman, Congregation Neve Shalom, St. Louis, Missouri

A s we discussed in the Introduction, two primary discoveries led us to develop a new model of treatment for individuals experiencing infertility. The first was that when we looked to the literature for guidance regarding effective treatment of these despairing clients, we found a remarkable absence of material written for the mental health practitioner. We therefore began treating our clients with infertility by using the traditional model for grief therapy and found that it was insufficient. Our second discovery was that, even though the usual treatment of infertility focused on resolution through parenting by adoption or using reproductive technologies, resolution of the infertility experience was not possible. These two discoveries caused us to listen to our own clients to see which treatment strategies contributed to healthy adjustment to the infertility diagnosis, and which strategies did not. What we heard helped us develop a new approach to treatment that specifically targeted our clients' loss of fertility.

Our new approach was created out of our work with clients who were functioning well despite their diagnosis. We discovered a critical distinction between the clients who were able to accommodate the loss of fertility and those who were not. We found that what determined how well clients adjusted to their diagnosis was the clients' ability to see that it was not the infertility itself but their *response* to the infertility that affected their functioning. Further, well-adjusted clients were able to integrate the *experience* of infertility into their identity. We have since learned how to facilitate this integrative process for our clients.

This chapter examines the different aspects of our new strategies for treatment: emphasizing that infertility is a condition; encouraging clients to acknowledge their loss; fostering client empowerment; and recognizing the impact of special concerns that may alter the course of therapy. In subsequent chapters we provide you with specific suggestions for using this model.

EMPHASIZING THAT INFERTILITY IS A CONDITION

When we ask our clients what issue they would like to address in therapy, "infertility" is the *only* one-word response we hear. People will provide elaborate details of their addiction issues, their marital problems, their parenting concerns, and their learning disabilities. In fact, clients initiating therapy for one of these reasons have been known to write complete paragraphs on our intake form. But when the one word *infertility* appears on the form, it conveys an entire constellation of issues that are associated with this perceived assault on our clients' lives. We have learned from conversations with our clients that the declaration "infertility" communicates that this is the single most pervasive issue in our client's life, and the most pervasive definition of his or her self. Thus, the primary objective of our model is to help clients stop labeling themselves as *infertile* and integrate the *experience* of infertility into their whole being, along with all other aspects of their identity.

Denying That Infertility Is a Definition of Self

As practitioners, we know that other aspects of our client's identity, such as their roles as professional and partner, are worthy of inquiry in a counseling session. In fact, those definitions of self, and an analysis of those definitions, are what ultimately facilitates the healing process. Other aspects of our client's identity, however, cannot be addressed until the client has grieved, mourned, and accepted his loss of the imagined biological child. The client is simply unable to even acknowledge that other definitions of his self are as integral to his being as is his sense of himself as "infertile."

The client's inability to see herself as a whole being illustrates her assumption that infertility has consumed her "former" self. We see this assumption expressed in such statements as "I was doing great before the infertility changed everything for me," or "I knew exactly who I was and what I wanted until the infertility took over." Thus, one of your primary tasks is to create an atmosphere of unconditional acceptance of all the aspects of your client's identity, emphasizing that the "former" self is still a part of her, and always was. This unconditional acceptance will help your client begin the process of restoring her sense of who she is. As your client reconnects with all aspects of her identity, you will see her translate your unconditional acceptance of her into unconditional acceptance of herself.

Acknowledging the Client as Expert

You can convey your unconditional acceptance of your client through a collaborative therapeutic relationship, as opposed to the traditional authoritative therapeutic relationship. We make a point of stating, early in the first session or in the discussion groups we lead, that we will be deferring to the client's expertise. We might say, for example, "Although we are here to listen and to guide you, we consider you to be the experts on the condition of infertility." This declaration equalizes the roles of the client and therapist, and gives clients an opportunity to take responsibility for influencing their own healing process. This is particularly important for clients who believe they have lost control over their destinies throughout the infertility treatment process.

Because of this perceived loss of control, it is critical that infertility counseling not provide solutions for clients but instead help individuals recognize and build on the strengths and coping mechanisms they already possess. However, these skills can be particularly difficult for clients to use if they have not yet understood that infertility is a condition and not a definition of self; their sense of self has been compromised by the experience of infertility. Therefore, we must be exceptionally astute listeners and observers in order to hear what clients reveal about themselves.

Clients tell us who they are through their dress, their choice of partners and friends, their body language, their interests, and their chosen professions. Although these forms of self-expression are not the primary focus of infertility counseling, they do provide you with useful information that helps you view your clients comprehensively. Close examination of your clients' choices also provides you with clues for how they problem solve and adapt in many areas of their lives. When you draw on these coping mechanisms to facilitate your client's healing, you honor him as the expert on himself, as he is the one who provides the solutions to the predicament.

In infertility counseling, we must be ever mindful that the client is the only authority on herself. This view is not usually shared by the other "experts" the client may have seen. We must also be able to reflect our client's expertise so that she is able to recognize her contribution to her own healing. If, for instance, you have a client who feels like a number, not a person, in his doctor's office, you could explore areas in his life where he felt valued. After discovering the ways in which he earned the respect of others, and applying those skills to his relationship with his doctor, you might say, "You have found it very helpful to explore your relationship with X. You have discovered ways to apply your ability to gain his respect to your relationship with your physician. I can see that you feel better about the course of your treatment, now that you have established a rapport with your doctor. Good going!" We cannot overemphasize how critical it is that our clients know that we know just how knowledgeable they are. We know of no other client population more motivated and determined to advocate on its own behalf. As you support this self-determination by helping your client accurately define himself and acknowledge that he is the expert on himself, you will facilitate his acceptance of the infertility diagnosis.

Promoting Acceptance of the Condition

A manifestation of the healing process is the client's acceptance of the entire self. We define acceptance as knowing how to be with and express one's feelings. It is normal in our culture to repress the feelings we define as negative, such as sadness, anger, frustration, and loneliness. This denial of feelings that we typically define as negative is particularly true for the client experiencing infertility because nothing has prepared her for the diagnosis or her response to it. Conversely, it is more appropriate in our culture to express the feelings we typically define as positive, such as feeling happy, excited, loving, and caring. The client's overall well-being depends on the client acknowledging and expressing *all* feelings. Clients experiencing infertility will be more likely to accept infertility as a condition if they are able to identify, acknowledge, and express their reactions to a condition that they were completely unprepared to accommodate. We highlight this lack of preparedness because the loss of fertility is an unanticipated loss, unlike the anticipated loss of a parent, or of a job upon retirement.

Clients can ultimately accept the unanticipated loss of fertility, or the condition of infertility, when they are able to stop defining themselves, their feelings, and their predicaments in terms of positive or negative and instead recognize and describe these things in factual terms. Our client Phoebe, who sought counseling after her third miscarriage, demonstrates how a client can acquire this perspective. We helped her see that her condition of infertility had nothing to do with her ability or inability to fulfill her identity roles as wife and daughter.

> After the second miscarriage, I just could not believe it. I kept thinking, "Why does this bad thing keep happening to me?" I take care of my body, I am pleasant in social situations, I am a great wife and daughter— Why wasn't all the good stuff I was being overriding the bad stuff in my life? Then, after the third miscarriage, it hit me: the good I was doing in life had nothing to do with the miscarriages. And once I realized that, I was able to see that the miscarriages meant my body simply did not hold the pregnancies. That was just the fact of the situation. That is all. It did not mean I was bad or that the miscarriages were a result of bad choices I had made. Then I was able to feel angry and sad, because I was no longer fighting my ill-defined fate. Before then, I could not even identify the sadness and anger because I was too busy trying to figure out why the good was not outweighing the bad, and what more good I could do to make that happen. I also realize now that I choose to be the wife and daughter that I am because that is just me. I do not do things because they are good; I do them because it is who I am.

When the process of promoting infertility as a condition is successful, and the client experiences a shift in perspective, he is able to see himself as a whole person with many aspects to his identity. He can then make the transition, for example, from defining himself as an "infertile person" to a person who has a condition called infertility.

A shift in perspective is the single most critical turning point in a client's journey toward the acceptance of infertility. Once they are able to see themselves as whole individuals, they are able to let go of the Why me? perspective that once dominated their thinking. It is as though they once believed that the infertility personally targeted them for an assault, and they subsequently awakened to the reality that the infertility had no idea within whose body it was residing. Furthermore, the infertility stops being a predator and becomes a condition, predicament, or situation. Our clients, as demonstrated by Phoebe, have described their new perspective as liberating. They report that they feel relieved to be able to get on with living their lives fully once again.

ENCOURAGING CLIENTS TO ACKNOWLEDGE THEIR LOSS

The most challenging aspect of the client's journey toward the acceptance of her infertility diagnosis is facing the losses associated with the diagnosis. These losses include the loss of the potential biological child and the loss of the opportunity to parent, which we explore in depth in Chapter Five. Facing these losses is exceptionally challenging because our culture fosters denial and encourages wishful thinking as appropriate means of facing situations we would rather not be in. Instead of expressing our sorrow over news we are not comfortable with, most of us want to make someone feel better and gloss over the truth. We say that our loved one "passed away" rather than "died" because it is less traumatic for us to pretend that our loved one is elsewhere rather than gone. And so it is with people experiencing infertility. There is a tendency for people to encourage the hope that "someday" it will all work out and that the individual will indeed experience biological parenting. This obvious avoidance of the situation can be confusing. The person is not only grieving in isolation but also at risk for feeling guilty and weak. It is as though the lack of acknowledgment for the loss reflects its unimportance or insignificance. Clients feel as though they should "get over it" or not feel the pain at all.

Because it is easier for both clients and practitioners to generate hope rather than to accept challenging predicaments, our treatment model provides concrete guidance for facing the losses associated with infertility, in the form of taking clients through the grieving process, giving them exercises, and helping them to develop rituals. The following discussion provides you with a theoretical foundation for how you can guide your clients.

Taking Clients Through the Grieving Process

As we discussed earlier, the loss of fertility is a loss that clients do not expect to endure. We must therefore be able to help our clients understand that their reactions to their infertility diagnosis are normal manifestations of their grief. We take clients through the grieving process by validating all their thoughts and feelings associated with their condition. Although this seems simple in theory, the grieving process is often hindered by the way in which clients compensate for the loss of fertility.

By *compensate* we refer to the tendency of some clients to pursue infertility treatment with vehemence. Sometimes the client's pursuit of medical treatment and the ensuing buildup of hope for a healthy pregnancy fosters denial of the condition and denial of the grief over the loss of the imagined biological child. In other words, clients can become so focused on infertility treatment that their grieving process is arrested. As a result, the grief reactions lie in wait, ready to be triggered at any time clients experience other losses.

Thus, a critical component of taking clients through the grieving process includes helping them manage their responses to the infertility treatment process and outcomes *in addition to* (rather than instead of) their responses to the diagnosis itself. We discuss the stages of grief and how you can specifically help your clients accommodate their losses in Chapter Five.

Giving Clients Exercises

We encourage our clients to keep journals, write letters, and write autobiographies (see Part Four), and we provide them with clear guidelines for doing these exercises to help them become more comfortable expressing themselves. Clients experiencing infertility often feel unable to express themselves because others do not know how to respond to their predicament. Sensing the discomfort in others, clients often deny their need to express what is happening to them. Written exercises are therefore useful because clients have the opportunity to experience their thoughts and feelings without relying on the involvement of another person. In addition, clients can experience writing on several different levels. Initially, there is the process of transforming thoughts into the written word. Clients are then able to see their thoughts and feelings, and hear them if they choose to read their writings out loud. Experiencing their feelings in numerous ways can provide the objectivity that was once missing from the client's perspective of their predicament. We believe that client writings create a figurative mirror with which clients can face their true self. Subsequently, our clients are able to identify their own progress patterns and cycles.

We have also developed tools that help clients see how all aspects of their identity hold equal significance to their whole being. Because clients often magnify the importance of infertility and at the same time minimize the significance of other life events, these tools allow clients to face their experience of infertility realistically. These tools (see Chapter Eleven) include the integrity wheel, a personal loss inventory, and affirmations. All of these exercises are designed to help clients shift their perspective from one of despair to one of seeing the possibilities available to them.

Helping Clients Develop Rituals

Rituals marking losses, such as funerals and memorial services for deaths and farewell parties for good-byes, are prominent in our culture. Because infertility is not an acknowledged loss in our culture, there are no rituals designed to recognize this loss. So we discuss with our clients the lack of prescribed rituals to mark the loss of a pregnancy or the loss of an imagined biological child. We encourage clients to design rituals that are meaningful for them. One client, George, shared the ritual he used every time his wife announced that her basal temperature took a nosedive after midmonth:

> I used to feel just rotten every time Gail turned over with that chart in her hands to tell me that she was not pregnant. She may as well have said, "You are not a real man," because that is what it meant to me month after month of no success. I got so tired of feeling so bad, I just knew there had to be a way of feeling good even though we could not get pregnant. In counseling I figured out that I always felt good about myself as a man when I did things that a lot of men do not think are manly, like cooking a special meal for Gail *and* doing the clean-up. So I decided that every morning when Gail told about another failed

attempt, I would first comfort her, maybe just hold her while she cried, but then I would call my boss and tell him I would be late because something important came up. Then I would go in the kitchen and make Gail a wonderful breakfast. One time I even picked flowers from the backyard and had them on the table for her. I have done this break-fast thing three times now, and even though it sounds like a gesture for my wife, and is good for her, too, I really do it for me. Gail tells me I am a woman's kind of man, and I really cannot think of any other kind of man I would rather be. We are still not pregnant, but at least now I have a ritual that reminds me I am still a man.

Once clients have created a ritual, they can use it repeatedly throughout the infertility treatment process. Some clients participate in their rituals at the end of each monthly cycle for which there is no pregnancy, as George demonstrated, and other clients have different rituals that mark lost pregnancies as well as failed treatments. Some of these rituals might include candle-lighting services, poetry read-ings, and demonstrations of self-care such as scheduling massages and workouts.

FOSTERING EMPOWERMENT

We express the concept of client empowerment through our efforts to foster the self-actualization of our clients. From our therapeutic per-spective, self-actualization is most clearly defined as the process of maximizing the client's individual potential. This process of self-actualization comprises the successful completion of tasks (pursuing educational paths, maintaining relationships, choosing a vocation) and the successful negotiation of the stages of life. Infertility presents clients with significant obstacles to making parenting one of their tasks during their negotiation of young adulthood (often referred to as "the childbearing years"). Thus one of the primary tasks of infertility coun-seling is to assist your clients in integrating their belief that parenting is essential to their self-actualization with the knowledge that infertil-ity may prevent them from having biological children.

In our practice, we address this challenge by exploring two funda-mental concepts: acceptance versus resolution and responsibility ver-sus control. In addition, we encourage self-advocacy as a means to powerful functioning.

Advocating Acceptance over Resolution

We originally began our work with couples experiencing infertility when we worked as adoption specialists doing prospective adoptive parent assessments (also known as home studies). We were instructed to make an assessment about whether or not these adoption applicants had made a healthy adjustment to their infertility diagnosis by determining if they felt they had resolved the infertility. Resolution of infertility was deemed a prerequisite to effective adoptive parenting. Thus, our instruction consistently equated the concept of resolution with a healthy adjustment to infertility. In our attempts to make this assessment and to understand what constituted resolution, we began to educate ourselves about this concept. When we thought about the word *resolution,* we thought about an ending, an absence of impact, or a solution to the problem. What we discovered was that although medical and other mental health issues could be resolved, when it came to infertility the emotional impact and sometimes its medical aspects could not be resolved.

Although we understood that resolution was a process, we were concerned by what this word implied to us and presumably to our clients. As we worked with couples throughout their attempts to parent and build a family, we frequently observed the reemergence of infertility issues, long after they had supposedly been resolved. We encountered parents who were still grieving the loss of the imagined biological child, couples in which the partners continued to resent each other for their individual responses to the infertility diagnosis, and clients who were never able to regain the spontaneity in their sexual relationship. (For a more in-depth discussion of these issues, see Chapters Five, Six, and Eight.)

Our observations and our clients' experiences led us to conclude that the idea that clients were supposed to put the infertility behind them and no longer suffer from its consequences encouraged a denial of the reality. It was at this point that we began advocating for acceptance instead of resolution. To us, acceptance indicates a state of *recognition.* Therefore, we now encourage our clients to recognize that infertility means loss and that this loss forever alters their self-image, their relationship with their partner, and their ideas about parenthood. We do not define a successful negotiation of the infertility experience as one that includes resolution. We talk about acceptance because acceptance means that our clients have passed through the initial stages of grief and have been able to grow from their experiences; the idea of acceptance more accurately describes what constitutes the healthy integration of infertility into a client's self-concept. A state of acceptance is also consistent with the behaviors and perspectives of the clients we counseled who seemed to be most at peace with the infertility experience.

Our clients have shown us that there are no magic time frames to follow, no magic words to hear, and no magic experiences to have (including biological parenting) that truly resolves the infertility experience. We therefore provide guidelines and ask questions that will foster acceptance of the infertility in whatever form is most comfortable for the client. For example, we do not offer answers and opinions about what acceptance is, but instead ask clients questions to help them discover what acceptance means to them. We might ask, "What options, besides biological parenting, do you feel you have for meeting your needs to nurture a child?" We are also convinced that even if resolution were possible, it would not be an optimal goal. True resolution requires a closure that prevents experiences from taking on new meaning in life. When clients remain open, they continue to grow. As this chapter's opening epigraph tells us, it is openness that facilitates the healing process, not cures, answers, and resolutions.

Promoting Responsibility over Control

An individual's potential can be affected by numerous conditions, such as physical impairments, oppression, socioeconomic status, sexism, and racism; a person's acknowledgment of these conditions is essential to her healthy functioning. This need to acknowledge their circumstances does not mean, however, that clients are powerless to change them. It does mean that clients must be firmly grounded in their present reality in order to appropriately *respond* to—take action regarding—their desire to change their circumstances. When clients respond to their desire for change or respond to an infertility diagnosis, they have choices about what form their responses take. Thus, we use the term *responsibility* to mean the ability to take action or the ability to respond to a given set of circumstances. That clients take a proactive stance toward their infertility diagnosis is central to our therapeutic approach.

Our conviction that true healing requires our clients to take action on their own behalf has played a key role in the development of our therapeutic methods. Often, it is a state of perceived powerlessness that prevents clients from addressing the situations in which they find themselves. The phrases "I feel powerless" and "I am out of control" are, in this culture, viewed as practically synonymous. The idea that being able to control a situation or a series of events and outcomes will serve as a solution to problems is a fallacy. What alleviates powerlessness is not control but the ability to take responsibility for how one reacts to the challenges and hardships in one's life. The following case illustrates a specific client's struggle with her feelings about her inability to control her own body and the application of our concepts to her situation.

Kevin and Diane had been married for six years and had been trying to get pregnant for three when Diane decided to seek infertility counseling. Diane was particularly concerned with the impact that infertility was having on her body image. She explained her concerns this way:

> I have always felt pretty good about how I looked—you know, healthy. Ever since we were diagnosed with undetermined fertility problems, I have been trying to figure out why *my* body does not work. I feel like I am out of touch with my physical self. I do not know my own body.
>
> I do not understand its strengths or limits or even if I can ever be comfortable with the way it looks again. I just do not feel like I am capable of anything physical. It is as if my body is out of my control and I have a screwed-up image of how I look—like you hear about with people who have eating disorders.

As Diane finished her story, she used the phrase "out of my control" to sum up her feelings. Throughout her explanation she talked about feeling incapacitated and being "out of touch." All these symptoms convey her feelings of disconnection from her body. To help her take responsibility for the actions she could take, we asked her questions that would lead her to pragmatic solutions.

For example, we asked Diane if there were any times or situations in which she felt more in tune with her body or more positive about her appearance. These questions helped Diane determine whether there were exceptions to the feelings she was describing; they also validated her concerns. Diane recalled a two-week period during the previous year when she had purchased and used a trial membership at a health club. She described how much she enjoyed swimming and using the weights, and thought this time period was probably an exception to the last three years.

In Diane's case we were able to determine that she would benefit from a regular exercise program that focused on strength and endurance. She felt that joining a health club that offered personal trainers would both meet her need to redevelop her awareness of her body's strengths and limitations and provide the structure and guidance she wanted.

This is a good example of how a therapist and client can explore the differences between control and responsibility. Diane felt she no longer had control over her own body or her thoughts about her body. In reality, Diane had not lost control of her body; she was reacting to the fact that her most basic *assumptions* about the functions of her body had been challenged. She was allowing the infertility diagnosis and the grief that accompanied the potential loss of biological parenting to seep into her overall attitude about her physical self. By exploring exceptions to her feelings, Diane realized she could take responsibility for change in her attitudes about her body. She recognized, for instance, that she could take responsibility for increasing her physical strength and her knowledge about how her body functions, and for shifting her attitude toward her ability to influence her overall physical health. This recognition is an important aspect of regaining influence over the infertility ordeal.

It is critical that clients understand their ability to influence their experience of infertility, because clients often report that the primary emotional consequence of the condition is the loss of control over reproduction and the decision of whether or not to become a parent. This perceived loss of control is in fact a misperception. Clients can have only relative degrees of control over their reproduction. They can influence reproduction through the decision to use birth control (which sometimes fails) or through abstinence from sexual activity. Ultimately, however, clients cannot have absolute control over conception unless they undergo an irrevocable medical procedure. Clients who receive an infertility diagnosis can, however, take responsibility for deciding how they will proceed and what they can do to alleviate some of their distress.

Our role as therapists is to empower clients to recognize that they can influence their response to their predicament. In other words, if we can educate, teach coping strategies, and facilitate clients' acceptance of their condition, clients can then make informed, proactive, and reality-based decisions. For clients to begin the process of healing through empowerment, they must recognize that reproduction is made up of a series of random events over which they have little *control* and some *influence.* Acknowledging this situation will reduce clients' frustration and possible disappointment and increase their chances of successfully taking responsibility for their emotional well-being.

As we have illustrated, client empowerment is a central theme in our approach. We believe that clients must first understand that achieving resolution and having control over infertility are not possible. Second, if clients can take a proactive stance toward the diagnosis and effects of infertility, they can begin to respond in ways that will further their self-actualization. Although clients may have little control over the challenges life presents to them, they do have tremendous influence over their response to those challenges. In this influence lies clients' true power.

We regularly share the following excerpt from *A Course in Miracles: A Return to Love,* by Marianne Williamson, with our clients because it conveys the power in taking responsibility for one's well-being. Because infertility can so thoroughly assault our clients' sense of who they are as men and women, and because our clients regularly tell us that they feel powerless and out of control, we want to remind them of how important it is for them to take part in their own healing. We also use the passage to remind ourselves that our clients have the intrinsic capacity to maximize their own potential and that we must use our skills to guide them toward that capacity.

> Our deepest fear is not that we are inadequate.
> Our deepest fear is that we are powerful beyond measure.
> It is not our darkness that most frightens us.
> We ask ourselves, who am I to be brilliant, gorgeous, talented and
>   fabulous?
> You are a child of God.
> Your playing small doesn't serve the world.
> There's nothing enlightened about shrinking so that other people
>   won't feel insecure around you.
> We were born to make manifest the glory of God that is within us.
> It's not just in some of us; it's in everyone.
> And as we let our own light shine,
>   we unconsciously give other people permission to do the same.
> And as we are liberated from our own fear
>   our presence automatically liberates others.

Encouraging Self-Advocacy

Clients gain the ability to advocate on their own behalf by gathering comprehensive information. Acquiring knowledge and thus gaining understanding is integral to the process of accepting the losses associated with infertility. Clients can acquire information through assigned reading, networking with others, and interviewing medical professionals. Through these experiences, as well as through discussions in therapy, clients learn how to talk with medical professionals, how to determine which treatments to pursue, and when to stop treatment. They also learn to define their own parameters—their comfort level—regarding what is disclosed to family and friends and what is and is not appropriate to discuss. They also learn when to look at adoption and child-free living, and how to manage finances. Chapter Eleven provides tools for these processes.

As the therapist you can promote self-advocacy by providing appropriate resources and referrals. (We discuss the importance of therapists' understanding resources in Chapter Two.)

Clients feel empowered when they access resources for themselves. Pauline told us:

> I feel so much better since I have begun to attend workshops. I go and listen to what the medical community is doing with new technology, I listen to adoptive parents talk about how they got their kids, and I even interviewed one couple who just decided not to have kids. Really knowing what my options were helped me to feel strong again. There was no way I could have faced the loss of my own baby until I knew I had choices. Now I do not feel like a whimpering fool incapable of making decisions for myself. Now I know who to talk to and how to talk to them. I still have no idea what I am going to do, but I know I am going to do something besides pray for my luck to change.

As you support your clients in their information-gathering process, you model what it takes to acknowledge difficult issues directly. Furthermore, you validate their experiences of devastation, frustration, and bewilderment when you provide explanations of how our culture deals with, and does not deal with, infertility. Acknowledging their loss allows clients to fully express the range of emotions they are experiencing.

RECOGNIZING AND TREATING
THE IMPACT OF SPECIAL CONCERNS

Both the client and the therapist may bring special concerns to therapy; these special concerns have a significant impact on the outcome of the therapeutic process.

Concerns Presented by Clients

In your assessment of clients who are experiencing infertility, you may identify issues that are unrelated to the infertility diagnosis but that nonetheless affect the ways in which your clients are coping with the infertility experience. You will need to acknowledge the existence of these issues and to recognize that they can significantly alter the course of infertility counseling. In later chapters we address several of the most prevalent issues that might influence the therapeutic process (you can also refer to the Special Concerns session in Chapter Ten); the following are some of the issues you may encounter:

- A history of being sexually assaulted
- Addictions (to drugs, alcohol, sex, or gambling)
- Cultural, racial, ethnic, and religious differences between clients and therapists
- Blended families

Any one or a combination of these issues will influence the client's therapeutic needs. You should address any special concerns as soon as you identify them, and incorporate them into the treatment plan. Your clients are your best resource for obtaining information about how an addiction to gambling or a particular religious belief has influenced their relationships, coping skills, perspectives about the infertility, or their grief reactions.

Furthermore, we strongly contend that it is perfectly appropriate for a therapist to acknowledge that she has little or no experience in dealing with a particular "special concern." Like the client, the therapist must be willing to educate herself and seek consultation for issues with which she feels unfamiliar. Because our theoretical framework relies on the client's expertise and education, and on his seeking solutions, an unfamiliar issue need not prohibit a successful outcome of therapy.

Concerns Presented by Therapists

Our limited formal education in infertility counseling has led us to rely on subjective sources in order to acquire information for effective treatment strategies. In the past, we looked to the lay community, as well as to therapists who have published their personal infertility stories for our information and education. Because these therapists are clearly experts on their *personal* experiences, however, they are the ones most challenged to maintain the client-as-expert perspective in their clinical practice.

Because these therapists, too, are their own infertility expert, prospective clients may perceive the power as lying outside themselves, which can instantly put them at a disadvantage. The following discussion highlights specific behaviors that therapists must exhibit in order to ensure a successful treatment outcome for their clients. The essential theme of these behaviors is that of maintaining appropriate boundaries.

The subject of setting boundaries is given great attention in the education of mental health professionals, and most therapists would agree that setting boundaries is fundamental in the therapeutic setting. However, we constantly encounter therapists who apparently disagree *in practice* with the "theory" that it is important to maintain boundaries between professionals and clients, at least when it comes to counseling clients who are experiencing infertility.

In the past ten years, we have attended dozens of conferences to supplement our education on infertility, adoption, and child-free living, and to maintain our licensure. In virtually every workshop and keynote address we have attended, at least one clinician has justified her expertise in the field through the telling of her *personal* experience with infertility. But in the same way that clients seek unbiased information from their therapists, at these conferences professionals want to gather unbiased information from their colleagues. We often wonder how these helping professionals judge the appropriateness of violating boundaries in the therapeutic setting.

We contend that helping professionals who *rely* on their personal experiences to teach and validate their expertise, whether in a workshop or in session with a client, have not established clear and ethical professional boundaries for themselves. The following is an example of a therapist who consistently demonstrates the blurring of personal and professional boundaries:

Seth and his wife were diagnosed with infertility and eventually decided to become parents through adoption. He currently works as a clinical psychologist specializing in infertility counseling. He is often asked to speak at workshops and regularly does so. The conference participants range from prospective adoptive parents to therapists who specialize in infertility counseling. Seth opens every seminar with *his* story of infertility, and various clients have reported that he begins initial therapy sessions in the same way. As he explains his experience, he generalizes his feelings and reactions to the experience of infertility for all people. He then projects that experience onto his definition of a healthy adjustment to an infertility diagnosis.

Conference evaluations consistently list Seth's talk as the least helpful portion of the seminar, and frequently recommend that it be eliminated from future conference schedules. Yet he continues to present at these conferences and continues to rely on his personal experience with infertility as the primary source of his expertise as a clinician who specializes in this field.

We find this trend quite disturbing. Primarily, we are concerned with the profession's willingness to endorse professionals simply because they have experienced infertility. We also are mystified by the general acceptance of self-disclosure as an educational tool. We find both of these practices—the acceptance of personal experience as objective information, and therapist self-disclosure—to be violations of professional boundaries. We have concluded that these boundaries are blurred because of the lack of available qualified infertility counselors. As we stated at the beginning of this section, therapists' lack of formal education about infertility seems to have caused all of us simply to take what we can get, and we are accepting subjective education through means that violate the ethical standards of our profession. Our clients need our expertise and our knowledge of what can actually help them, not our personal stories. We believe that we are truly able to help others only when we no longer need our own story to justify our ability to help. We therefore recommend that therapists refrain from self-disclosure and heal themselves prior to engaging in a therapeutic relationship with others who are experiencing infertility.

REFRAINING FROM SELF-DISCLOSURE.   Clients experiencing infertility often struggle with feelings of powerlessness. Those feelings can be compounded when therapists disclose personal experiences related to their own infertility ordeal. Any self-disclosure on the therapist's part can leave the therapist wide open for such comments as "How can you understand? Your experience isn't the same," or "Who are we talking about here, anyway?" Furthermore, therapist self-disclosure can make the client feel obligated to take care of the therapist, and it is not the client's responsibility or role to do this. We have an ethical obligation to be aware of our own issues so that we do not provide personal accounts masquerading as objectivity.

We do agree, however, that it can be helpful to share one's experience with others who have had the same challenge. Support groups, such as the national organization RESOLVE, can fulfill this function. Friends and compassionate family members can also meet this need. We strongly encourage clients experiencing infertility to seek others with whom they can commiserate.

HEALING THYSELF, FIRST. Worst of all are the professionals who unconsciously use clients and the issues they share as a means to process their own issues. In this situation, practitioners may foster client self-absorption and prohibit a client from moving beyond a phase in healing that the practitioner may still be stuck in. The admonition, *Physician, heal thyself,* is appropriate here, as those who most need help often end up helping others. We feel it is critical to take an honest look at yourself to determine how well you, the practitioner, have integrated your infertility experience. If you are a therapist who has effectively integrated your experience and see it in context with your identity, it is possible that you can be effective in counseling others who have also experienced infertility. We believe, however, that it is more appropriate to counsel people with infertility on a random basis, as opposed to actively pursuing the "infertile population" as consumers of your counseling practice. This pursuit would evidence lack of integration of the issue; in other words, it would be a sign that "infertility" is *your* one-word answer to the question, What issue would you like to address in therapy? It is simply too pervasive in *your* life. And as long as this is the case, your clients are at risk for not getting the services they sorely need.

A good test to help you determine whether or not you have integrated your own infertility experience is to notice whether your clients trigger memories of your infertility experience. If your memories are triggered, and you subsequently find your attention on your own past, then you cannot be completely present for your client. Thus, you are probably better suited to the role of compassionate peer rather than the role of professional therapist. Only when genuine healing takes place can we expect the experiences of our personal losses to be fully integrated into our identities. Only then can we offer our clients a model of what it is to stand in acceptance of the predicaments that shape our lives.

—⁓—

As Rabbi Goodman's insightful quotation at the opening of the chapter suggests, we heal through the process of opening up, not closing down. Our new model of infertility treatment honors this path for healing through acknowledging the client as expert, promoting self-acceptance over self-absorption, providing support and education, and remaining honest with ourselves by assessing on an ongoing basis who the best helper is for the clients who have trusted us with their deepest selves during the life-altering experience of infertility. We now move on to discuss the concrete skills we must bring to the therapeutic process in order to facilitate our clients' healing journeys.

CHAPTER TWO

Learning the Essential Skills of Infertility Counseling

The Master said, "You, shall I teach you what knowledge is? When you know a thing, to recognize that you know it, and when you do not know a thing, to recognize that you do not know it. That is knowledge."

—*Confucius*, Analects

Before you can expect your clients to take specific actions to heal themselves, you have to know how to guide them safely through the infertility experience. Our clients need skilled guidance because healing requires a change in perspective and coping methods, and change is difficult. Although most clients understandably deny that they are reluctant to change, it is natural for everyone to resist change. Dieters in the initial stages of a new diet, for example, often keep weight on or actually gain additional weight. A physiological response in the dieter's body fights to maintain the original weight in order to ensure the body's survival. And so it is with behavioral changes: the subconscious fights to maintain the status quo. Individuals look for reasons why new suggestions will not work, or they try them halfheartedly so that they are doomed to fail.

Because it is natural for human beings to resist change, therapists must provide support that is gentle as well as challenging. You can initiate supportive conversation by asking clients to discuss matters that are not related to the infertility experience. We find that clients particularly enjoy talking about their successes, especially about how they arrive at success. When they are able to grasp exactly which behaviors produce successful outcomes, clients are then able to transfer these behaviors to areas in their lives with which they are struggling. Clients are thus able to discover that they already have what it takes to improve their functioning during all the stages of the infertility experience. But we cannot facilitate our clients' discovery of these skills unless we are intentional about it. We must know how to apply our therapeutic skills to the unique experience of infertility.

As therapists, we acquire some skills naturally but must learn to develop others. We must thoroughly examine and understand all the skills we possess before we use them in the therapeutic setting. Even though some skills appear to be basic, their effective use is crucial when we counsel clients who feel powerless. This chapter explores communication skills and guiding skills. Our demonstration of these skills as they relate to infertility counseling will enable you to help your clients rebuild their identities and effectively manage the specific challenges they face throughout the infertility ordeal.

COMMUNICATION SKILLS

Effective coping throughout the infertility ordeal demands good communication between partners and between client and therapist. The skills discussed in this section—expressing warmth and compassion, demonstrating empathy, providing reflective listening, remaining silent, and avoiding erroneous assumptions—are classified as communication skills because they involve *listening* and *responding* to your clients. Well-developed communication skills are critical for effective infertility counseling, and we discuss them here for the benefit of new therapists or therapists who have little or no experience in infertility counseling.

Expressing Warmth and Compassion

Webster's New World Dictionary of American English defines *warmth* as "the quality or state of being warm in feeling—to infuse with a feeling of . . . well being," and *compassion* as "sorrow for the . . . trouble of another or others, accompanied by an urge to help." As a therapeutic skill, conveying warmth and compassion requires both appropriate and authentic expressions of these sentiments. Along with empathy, the ability to demonstrate warmth and convey compassion constitute the foundation of every effective therapeutic relationship, irrespective of the therapeutic issue, be it infertility, sexual abuse, or chemical dependency.

DEMONSTRATING WARMTH.   In working with clients who have experienced infertility, we have found that expressing warmth is essential to building our clients' trust in us. Many of our clients tell us that the impersonal nature of medical treatment for infertility leaves them feeling like nameless, faceless laboratory animals. We do not want the therapeutic experience to leave clients feeling the same way, so we show our clients that we care about them as individuals. We do this because we do care, and also to convey that we have our clients' best interests at heart.

We show that we care for our clients through our gestures, facial expressions, and posture, and through our expressions of respect for the client's views, feelings, and perspectives. Our body language and verbalizations reflect our willingness to accept the client, indicate that we are listening, and encourage the client to continue to express herself. These behaviors are supportive. They are not intended to convey our opinion of what the client says and does but our appreciation of the client's perspective, simply because it is a part of the client.

CONVEYING COMPASSION.   Compassion is also essential to developing trust between therapists and clients. Compassion is the expression of warmth coupled with the intention to act. Compassion is without judgment and prevents our making inauspicious judgments about a client's situation. Compassion allows us to see our clients' unhealthy behaviors and chaotic circumstances as *symptoms* of their distress. Having compassion for our clients means that we have genuine regard for them and believe that their distress is real and understandable. By acknowledging clients' distress in this way, we show that we are engaged in problem solving rather than in an effort to learn how our clients may be to blame for their distress. In infertility counseling the distinction between acknowledging and blaming is an important one, because we have found that our clients often blame themselves for their infertility.

When clients are not able to have a biological child, they often internalize their biological "shortcomings" into their self-concept. Our clients may begin to feel as though the infertility is symbolic of their unsuitability for parenthood. When we demonstrate compassion for our clients' feelings and experiences, we are telling them that they are valuable. When we take the focus off of the client as the cause of the problem and focus on the fertility issues, we normalize our clients' feelings about their experience with infertility. Although compassion alone will not sustain an effective therapeutic relationship, a therapeutic relationship without compassion will not sustain the client.

Demonstrating Empathy

Like warmth and compassion, empathy is particularly helpful to clients in infertility counseling. This is because clients experiencing infertility often feel isolated from the broader culture, and they need to know that we understand their pain. Being empathic is what gives us credibility and helps our clients listen to and trust what we have to say. But being empathic can be challenging for us, because we cannot demonstrate empathy without projecting our own feelings onto our clients. We must be able to move beyond this projection in order to help our clients.

RECOGNIZING PROJECTION IN THE THERAPEUTIC RELATIONSHIP.   We are projecting when, for example, we remember *our* sadness over a lost dream and assume we know our clients' sadness when *their* dream (of the biological child) is lost. Although our ability to access our own memories of loss and to reconnect to the feelings associated with those memories may help us better understand our clients, it does not mean that we share their pain. *Sharing pain* means we are experiencing someone else's pain as though it were our own pain. If we do share our clients' pain, we risk getting lost in the details of the shared memory of the experiences and in the emotions related to the experiences. It is not the projection of our feelings that is beneficial to our clients but our ability to express the *outcome* of the projection, which is our warmth and compassion, that will help our clients.

This distinction between the projection of our feelings and the outcome of the projection is confusing. When we only project, we are too connected to ourselves, in that moment, to express genuine warmth and compassion. What is required in the therapeutic relationship is to step outside of ourselves to gain perspective. When we do this, we are able to display warmth and compassion. This confusion explains why we see in the current literature on infertility counseling such a broad misuse and overemphasizing of empathy as the primary therapeutic tool: it is easier to dwell in the development of empathy (projecting our own feelings) than it is to exhibit the outcome of empathy (warmth and compassion).

DISTINGUISHING EMPATHY FROM SYMPATHY.   No matter how analogous your situation may seem to that of your client, the situations are different. In addition, it is not necessary for you to have experienced infertility in order to be empathic about the infertility experience. Without the ability to distinguish between our clients' experiences and our own, we cannot have an objective perspective on the client's reactions to a given circumstance. Overidentification with our clients causes us to assume that their infertility experience mirrors our own and the experience of everyone else who has struggled with infertility. Remembering that all individuals are unique helps us acknowledge to our clients that their experience of infertility is unique. Maintaining this distinction between empathy and sympathy is what facilitates our therapeutic effectiveness and allows our clients to trust that we will provide something they are not getting in any of their other relationships. When we maintain this therapeutic distance we are also preventing the blurring of professional boundaries.

Although the concept of maintaining distance may seem incongruent with the concept of empathy, genuine empathy *requires* distance. One might wonder, How can I be empathic if I am distant? We assert that empathy without distance is actually sympathy. *Sympathy* is defined as a mutual understanding that arises from feeling the same way as someone else does. It is very clear to us that sympathy does not belong in the therapeutic relationship and is actually empathy in suspended development. Without distance from our clients' experiences we have the same ability to be objective with them as we would have with ourselves: very little. Once we are free of the entanglement of our personal experiences, the state of being empathic acts as a catalyst allowing us to "open our eyes" and see our clients for who they *are,* rather than who we *think* they are.

Providing Reflective Listening

Clients experiencing infertility often feel as if no one understands what they are going through. Our clients report that doctors and other professionals with whom they consult often tell them what they should be doing instead of listening to what they want to do. Because our clients' need to be heard is so profound, we must be able to provide them with reflective listening throughout their experience with infertility.

Listening can be difficult, however. Some therapists practice reflective listening by stating, "I hear you saying . . . ," followed by a restatement of the client's own words. Although there is value in this literal approach, some clients report that they perceive it as insulting and a waste of their time to hear "my own words thrown back in my face." Clients instinctively know that anyone can repeat the words they have spoken and that it does not mean their words have actually been *heard*. We have found it helpful to let our clients hear themselves in *our* words so that they can be assured that we have heard, processed, and received what they have said. The following dialogue illustrates our approach to reflective listening.

CLIENT: I am scared I am going to come unglued over all this infertility stuff.

THERAPIST: You are afraid you are falling apart.

CLIENT: Yes! And I cannot do that because my wife depends on me to be whole.

THERAPIST: Are you saying that you think you would be letting your wife down if you were not all in one piece?

CLIENT: Oh, I know I would be letting her down. I am her rock. And rocks do not fall apart.

THERAPIST: At least not this rock.

CLIENT: Right. Not me. I have got to keep it together for her.

THERAPIST: It sounds like you are pretty clear about what your wife expects from you. Would you be willing to double-check this with her?

CLIENT: You bet I would. Maybe she will give me a break.

This client demonstrated a willingness to shift from holding his original position—that his wife would not let him fall apart—to considering that she just might. We assert that he was open to a new possibility because he was heard. When clients do not feel heard, they may feel the need to defend their position. Defensive clients shut down and are unwilling to receive new information. When clients shut down, we have no chance of reaching them with suggestions.

Reflective listening also requires us to refrain from interpreting, analyzing, or challenging what our clients say. When we assume we know what clients mean or we analyze clients, we are usually motivated by something other than the will to listen. Perhaps it is our desire to have our client see himself in a different light, or a wish that he could change his victim stance. Whatever the motivation, we must realize that when we assume we know what our clients mean we are motivated by *our* agenda and not our clients'. Speaking out of our agenda alienates and confuses clients and can prevent them from progressing in therapy. Only when clients *feel* heard, not merely when we *convey* that they have been, are they able to reconsider their position and move forward.

Remaining Silent

Genuine listening also requires our knowing when *not* to speak. Although you will sometimes find it difficult to do so, remaining silent while a client is thinking is a basic therapeutic tool. The ability to remain silent is critical in infertility counseling, because our clients are used to having their predicament spark nervous chatter from others who do not know how to respond to their despair. Clients experiencing infertility frequently tell us that they have been told by so many professionals what they should be doing that it is refreshing when a professional just listens to what *they* have to say. Therefore, we must strive to recognize our clients' nonverbal signals that they are searching for the right words, and learn to be comfortable with the silence that is a normal part of this process.

Because it is a natural human response to "fill up" the space with our own thoughts, we can fall into expressing our clients' thoughts for them. When we do our clients' thinking and speaking for them, we run the risk of being inaccurate as well as annoying to our clients. When we interrupt our clients' thoughts we do not allow them the time to process their thoughts in their own time. We must not interrupt our client's train of thought for the sake of easing our discomfort. When we are uncomfortable, it is our responsibility to manage that discomfort in silence, or we risk forgetting that the session belongs to the clients, for their agenda, on their terms. Remaining aware of who "owns" the session is especially important in infertility counseling because so much of our clients' experience with infertility engenders feelings of powerlessness. Clearly, if we are uncomfortable with silence, if we interrupt our clients, speak for them, finish their sentences, we will only be exacerbating that sense of powerlessness.

You can manage your discomfort during long periods of silence by using self-talk. You might remind yourself to "be patient," "wait," or simply "shut up!" You can do this very quickly so you do not lose your focus on the matter being discussed. During the silence, you can use the time to observe your client's body posture and facial expressions. If your client appears to be visibly uncomfortable you might softly encourage her by saying, "Take your time." Even when she does not speak, she is communicating information. Silence also affords you the opportunity to get back on track, if you have drifted, so that you are fully present when your client does begin to speak.

When we remain silent, we are also modeling the skill for couples. This modeling teaches clients how to be silent for each other. Remaining silent and allowing a partner to continue talking and thinking demonstrates a genuine commitment to improved communication. This commitment is critical because most of the problems we see between couples who are struggling with infertility are manifestations of ineffective communication. We believe that when partners honor silence-while-thinking, they express respect for the unique ways in which people process their thoughts and ideas.

Avoiding Erroneous Assumptions

Both clients and therapists make assumptions. In infertility counseling, understanding the role of assumptions is critical because you as a therapist will invariably make them and behave according to them. And you cannot help your clients if you believe something to be true when in fact it is not. It is ultimately your responsibility to acknowledge your assumptions so that you can determine exactly what information you are filtering in and what information you are filtering out during therapy sessions. If you allow your assumptions to go unchecked, it is possible for you and your client to engage in two entirely different conversations and not even know it.

Your clients also make assumptions about the things you say and about the meaning that events have in their lives. An ancient Jewish folktale illustrates the power of assumptions, and how unchecked beliefs influence one's behavior. It also illustrates a common approach to life, irrespective of a specific predicament such as an infertility diagnosis.

There once was a poor old Jewish man named Yenkl. He worked hard his entire life, serving God and providing for his family. Though he had very few material possessions he felt satisfied that his life was honorable. One day, when he was very tired and weak, he learned that a distant relative had died and left him a small fortune. He decided that the first thing he wanted to do was go to a nice restaurant. There he ordered a divine meal, not worrying about the cost, and enjoyed his leisure immensely. When he finished his meal he began to hobble out of the restaurant. He then glimpsed the tailor's shop across the way and decided he should have a fine suit! Never had he owned such a wondrous garment. As he crossed the street, a horse and carriage came in his path, and Yenkl was struck and instantly killed. Later, in heaven, he asked, "Why, God? I spent my entire life serving you, doing as you wished. Was one day of good fortune too much to ask?" Throwing up his hands, God replied, "Yenkl, Yenkl, Yenkl! I did not know it was you!"

Like Yenkl, many clients experiencing infertility assume that what is happening *to* them is *about* them. In this story, Yenkl assumes that a lifetime of service to God will ultimately be appreciated by God. Yenkl assumes that God is the divine master of Yenkl's fate. When God replies that He was not even aware that it was Yenkl who (1) received the good fortune, or (2) was struck by a horse and carriage, or (3) led a life of good will (we provide several choices here, lest we ourselves be guilty of assuming what it was that God meant by the statement, "I did not know it was you!"), we can instantly see that Yenkl's assumptions are indeed inaccurate.

Yenkl's assumptions may very well have been the driving force behind how he chose to live his life, and they caused him to behave in an accusatory manner toward God. But it seems clear to us that Yenkl's bad fortune—being killed after so little time to enjoy his new wealth—was *not about him.* In other words, Yenkl's bad fortune, like a client's infertility, was probably a result of several variables instead of something Yenkl did or did not do. There is nothing in the story indicating that God had a master plan for Yenkl, only that Yenkl *assumed* He did. Some clients assume that their infertility experience is part of a divine plan and that if they can figure out what God is trying to tell them, they may be able to alter their fate. If Yenkl had known that his assumptions were inaccurate, he probably would have behaved differently toward God. Yenkl might also have made other choices for his life had he held a completely different set of assumptions. We share this tale with clients who assume that their infertility diagnosis can be altered through specific behaviors (that are not related to medical intervention).

Clients who experience infertility are liberated by the idea that the infertility is not about them and not necessarily a result of something they did or did not do. When our clients shed the assumption that infertility is a personal assault, they realize they are free to influence their responses in each phase of the infertility experience.

Rather than assuming that you know what your client is trying to tell you, and possibly making erroneous assumptions, you must remember to ask your clients to tell you exactly what they mean when they speak. When we voice our assumptions, we provide ourselves opportunities to have our inaccurate assumptions corrected (as Yenkl did). We also model for our clients how to free themselves of harmful assumptions or of those that take away their power to make clear choices for themselves.

GUIDING SKILLS

Guiding skills complete the repertoire of skills integral to infertility counseling. Guiding skills include reframing situations, augmenting perspective and context, using metaphors and analogies, using pragmatic problem-solving, and providing relevant resources.

Reframing Situations

Individuals experiencing infertility often feel desperate, hopeless, or utterly lost and without direction. They unconsciously use absolutes—*always, never, forever*—in their statements. Absolutes prevent people from seeing the things that *are* working in their lives, and consequently contribute to the sense of despair clients experience. It is thus our job as therapists to help eradicate the absolutes and reframe them with more realistic descriptions—*sometimes, usually, occasionally.*

In reframing, we suggest numerous ways in which clients can see a situation. We have found that a powerful way to do this is by seeing clients as who they could be as opposed to the troubled "infertile" individuals they present when initiating therapy. One of our mottos is "Treat people as though they are who they could be." We heard this statement at a Viktor Frankl workshop and have it posted in our office so that we can be ever mindful of its message.

Clients do not seek help from mental health professionals when they feel that things are going well in their lives. In fact, people struggling with infertility are in crisis when they come through our doors. They often claim that they are at a breaking point and express that they "cannot go on this way much longer." We have learned that reframing our clients' situation can serve to build them up from their place of despair.

USING REFRAMING TO EMPOWER. When you treat clients as though they already are who they could be, your language shows that you see not simply a person facing the challenges that infertility brings but also a person with strengths. Seeing your clients as complete individuals with traits that do and do not empower them emphasizes that clients are not their problems but instead are people *with* problems. Holding on to this basic tenet enables you to ask questions that guide you into the arenas in your clients' lives where things *are* working for them.

A couple experiencing infertility may find it natural to say, for example, that without children their lives have no meaning. If you question both partners about their professions, though, and they are able to speak with excitement about the contributions they make in their daily work, they may be able to see meaning in their lives regardless of whether or not they have an opportunity to parent. By helping your clients reframe their ideas of what constitutes a meaningful life, you can help them move toward their future optimistically, despite their infertility experience. It is important to request that clients stretch beyond their usual way of thinking, because new possibilities and solutions for the original problem (in this case, being childless) may come to light for them.

The case of Tim and Leeann, who had been struggling with infertility for seven years, illustrates how you can guide your clients to see their strengths by helping them reframe their situation.

TIM: I do not know what to do anymore. I feel like a complete failure. Nothing seems to be going right for us.

LEEANN: I feel that way, too. The treatments are not working, and I am miserable all the time.

TIM: We want our old lives back. Back when we did not have so many problems.

THERAPIST: What was going on in your lives when you felt there were no problems?

LEEANN: Well, for one, we had not decided to start a family yet. We went to work every day, came home, talked about our days, and spent a lot of time together.

TIM: We pretty much did whatever we wanted. We had money in the bank and went on trips whenever we wanted. Now, we have no money and no time to just do what we like to do. We had everything managed.

THERAPIST: What is happening in the time you used to spend with one another?

LEEANN: Doctors' appointments and a lot of down time at night just feeling bad.

THERAPIST: It sounds like you still have time to be together but are perhaps too drained at the end of your day to do anything.

TIM: Yes, that is true.

THERAPIST: It seems that although the circumstances in your lives may have changed, the two of you are still the same two people with the same interests.

From this point, we went on to recommend that Tim and Leeann schedule nights with one another after work the way they once did. By refusing to focus on the belief that "nothing" was going right for them, we treated Tim and Leeann like the high-functioning, every-thing-managed people they once saw themselves to be.

USING CAUTION WHEN REFRAMING.   We caution you, however, that there is a risk involved in reframing clients' situations and treating clients as though they are who they could be. The risk is that we may project *our* ideas of who our clients are and how they could view their situation. In the case of Tim and Leeann, if we had suggested that they see their spare time as an opportunity to enjoy being together, they might have responded with frustration, anger, or both. They could have justifiably wondered if we had even heard how drained they were. Instead, we pointed out that their interests seemed unchanged since the infertility diagnosis. Thus they are responsible for deciding how and when to pursue their interests.

Clearly, we do not want to minimize the problems our client's are experiencing. Instead, by listening, validating, and establishing trust, we can effectively reframe our client's experience of infertility. By demonstrating that we can see what the client once saw in herself, we make the goal of rediscovering the client's original self believable and obtainable. Once the client acquires an awareness of her original self, she will be in a better position to broaden her perspective about the infertility.

Augmenting Perspective and Context

For clients to accept a diagnosis of infertility and learn to cope with the implications of the diagnosis, they often need to gain a broader perspective—gain distance—on the problem. Distance can come from seeking an objective opinion or just allowing the initial shock of an unexpected occurrence to wear off. Because an infertility diagnosis can affect many areas of our client's life, he can find it very difficult to step outside his own situation and gain a new perspective. Our clients often tell us that it seems as though living their daily lives has become secondary to dealing with the infertility diagnosis.

FINDING A MANAGEABLE PERSPECTIVE.   As therapists, it is our job to assist clients in putting the infertility into a more manageable perspective. We try to help them see the infertility as a manageable problem that can be addressed in a step-by-step process: we can take each issue, examine it, and then move on to the next issue or step. We also relate infertility and our clients' reactions to their diagnosis to cultural norms and gender, and to clients' own attitudes and belief system. For instance, if clients believe that adoption is not a viable alternative for them because of financial constraints, we educate them about the various money-saving alternatives that are available. We discuss employer reimbursement programs, adoption tax credits, and organizations that offer low-interest loans to adoptive parents.

Another example would be a client who believes that she must carry and give birth to a child in order to bond with that child. We would talk about all the behaviors and interactions that facilitate bonding *after* a child is born. We might compare the development of a parent-child relationship to the relationship she has with her life partner. We often tell clients that we do not have to know our life partners from the moment of conception in order to develop a loving and caring relationship with them. We do acknowledge, however, that relationships between adoptive children and their parents are different from relationships between biological parents and children, but only because they are developed under different circumstances. The intensity and strength of the relationship is dependent not on biology but on a genuine desire to facilitate and maintain the attachment between themselves and the child.

FINDING AN APPROPRIATE CONTEXT.   Many of the clients we see in our practice report that they feel isolated and that no one understands how much the infertility diagnosis has affected them. Clients often tell us they feel as though they should just be able to get past the infertility, to move on. Our clients also stress their desire to "rid themselves of the pain and frustration" associated with their diagnosis, and they do not understand "why they can't stop feeling depressed." They report perceiving that other people in their lives are also wondering when they are going to stop letting the infertility rule their existence. This dynamic is often also being played out in the marriage: one partner is frustrated with the other partner's inability to focus on anything other than the infertility and the infertility treatment.

As we counsel clients about these feelings, we begin by discussing infertility in the context of loss (loss of reproductive freedom, of the biological child, of privacy, and so on). We stress that acceptance of these losses is a process, not an event. It takes time and the support of others to begin to feel "normal" again. The key is for our clients to allow themselves that time and to seek support from others (family, friends, a support group) who understand the nature of the loss. By placing infertility in the context of loss, clients are usually, over time, able to accept their reaction as valid. They may choose to change some of their coping mechanisms, but clients then recognize that there is a difference between a grief response and being "crazy." (We explore loss and grief more fully in Chapter Five.)

A significant number of your clients may already recognize that infertility is a loss when they begin the counseling process. However, they may still be struggling with the amount of time it is taking them to feel better or less out of control. Again, you may need to help them put infertility into a context that allows them to see that they are attempting to manage their infertility diagnosis in a fertility-focused world. You can discuss the prevalence of cultural messages that emphasize the joys and fulfillment that come from pregnancy, childbirth, children, and parenting. You can discuss the messages that emphasize the disappointments and emptiness that come from being single, childless, and career-focused (instead of family-focused). You can remind them of our society's tendency to be hard on people who are unsuccessful at whatever it is they are attempting to do, not to mention the cultural messages that blame lack of success on lack of determination and motivation. (We discuss the relationship between cultural messages and infertility more fully in Chapter Five.)

As we have previously discussed, your clients may also have lost sight of who they were before they were diagnosed as "infertile." They may be unable to see themselves as people who are experiencing infertility, but instead see themselves only through the filter of their diagnosis. In these situations, we strive to assist our clients in placing the infertility into the context of their entire being—in seeing that infertility is only one part of their whole identity. In working through these issues, we ask clients to complete exercises (see Chapter Eleven) that can help them clarify the roles they play in their life, their personality characteristics, their values, and their life goals.

When your client is able to see the experience of infertility as a part and not the whole of herself, her perspective on the infertility changes. The infertility is no longer as big or as powerful as it once was; it is still influential, but it is no longer formidable. One of our clients summed up this concept:

> I used to feel like I was walking around with a neon sign on my head that said "Hi, I'm infertile." Not "My name is Janice," or "I am a real estate agent," but "I'm infertile." I felt like everywhere I turned I was confronted by a reminder of the infertility and that it was written all over me. When I was finally able to look at the infertility and see it as an experience that ultimately made me a more compassionate and grateful person, it just did not seem so big anymore. I realized that I had survived a devastating experience and that I had dealt with it pretty well. I am not saying I am grateful for the experience, but I am grateful for what it taught me about myself: that I am strong and that I have a lot of things in my life that make me who I am. Some of those things, like being strong and successful, are what helped me to come out of this with a clearer sense of who I am, and what is important to me.

Using Metaphors and Analogies

Because everyone's life experience is unique, we cannot assume that we understand the points our clients make, nor can we assume our clients are able to identify with the points we are trying to make. It is therefore helpful to develop a repertoire of metaphors and analogies to ensure effective communication.

We often find ourselves saying, "It's like when . . ." A client may feel overwhelmed by a particular emotion, and in order to anchor him to something broader than his personal experience we will say, "It's like when . . ." The following case shows how a metaphor helped Jim view the affects of his infertility from a different perspective.

JIM: Everything revolves around our infertility. We cannot go to baby showers because Cindy will fall apart. We cannot have sex tonight because we had it last night. We cannot go to Europe this summer because the new procedure will take the savings. We cannot talk to most of our friends because they all have kids and we will just get depressed. I just feel like checking out; I cannot stand it anymore. Do you know what I am getting at?

THERAPIST: It's like when you turn on the news and it seems that all they are reporting on is deaths. Then you turn the station and the next report is about someone who got murdered. You just keep channel-surfing looking for something other than news stories about deaths.

JIM: Yes! It's like everywhere I turn the infertility is hitting me in the face!

THERAPIST: Eventually, you do find *real* news where they are talking about many current events.

JIM: So, it may take awhile to find a station that really reports the news, but there is one out there.

THERAPIST: Yes, I think that is true.

JIM: I just need to keep turning the channels, and I will find something in my marriage that is not about infertility.

The use of the news as a metaphor for the way Jim was feeling about his marriage was particularly helpful for him. Through this metaphor he was able to see that there are many things in life that appear to be imbalanced but are not, necessarily. And he was able to see that, like the news that does not *really* just report murders and deaths, his marriage was not *really* just about infertility. Acquiring this kind of perspective can help diminish a client's confusion about his predicament.

We repeatedly hear the question, "Do you know what I mean?" Often clients will ask this after they have provided an explanation or description. Although clients sometimes unconsciously blurt out this question in attempt to seek validation, we assert that our clients genuinely want to know if we understand what they've just said. We are in the habit of automatically saying, "I am not sure. Explain it to me another way." This response encourages the client to consider analogies or metaphors that will help us "know what they mean," affording them the opportunity to sort out their thoughts and consider how they are communicating them. Again, as you model the use of metaphors and analogies, your clients gain tools to improve intimate relationships outside the therapeutic relationship.

Volumes have been written on the use of metaphors and analogies in therapy. Appendix A provides a suggested reading list for further exploration of the subject. The following is a list of several of the metaphors we have found most useful for our clients.

- Undergoing infertility treatment is like a big gamble: you keep paying your money in the hopes that you will win and get pregnant.

- Ongoing infertility treatment is like an addiction: you keep hoping for the thrill of a pregnancy to save you from your despair.

- The all-consuming nature of the infertility experience is like that of the experience of losing someone you love: in both experiences, you cannot believe the world is going on around you as though there is nothing profound occurring.

- Reinitiating medical intervention because a new technology has emerged is like returning to the blackjack table simply because the dealer has changed.

- Scheduling sex is like scheduling time to go to the bathroom.

- The paper chase in international adoption is like trying to buy and sell a house at the same time: there are so many people and variables involved in order to pull it off, it is inevitable that something will go wrong.

We have found that the best way to learn which metaphors and analogies will work comes from listening to your clients. You can also use their professions, skills, hobbies, and relationships to draw on so that the metaphors you use will be meaningful for them.

Using Pragmatic Problem Solving

The aftermath of an infertility diagnosis is marked by a need to make concrete decisions during an emotional time. Clients seeking the help of counseling professionals during this time are usually feeling vulnerable and overwhelmed by the diagnosis and its implications. Our clients consistently report that what they most need during this time is help with sorting out all the various issues associated with the infertility diagnosis. Our approach to meeting this need is to model a practical, step-by-step approach to problem solving and to encourage clients to use it themselves.

MAKING DECISIONS USING A PRAGMATIC APPROACH.   Initially, clients are often faced with making decisions regarding medical options and the course of treatment. They need to make decisions about whether or not to pursue medical treatment, who will provide the treatment, where to go for their treatment, how much they can afford to spend, and what types of treatment are appropriate (morally, medically, and financially) for them to pursue. Clients are making all these decisions in conjunction with their attempt to manage the emotional aspects of the infertility diagnosis. It is a time of crisis (we define crisis as a turning point marked by emotional distress and increased demands on the time and energy of those involved), which calls for crisis management.

When our clients are in crisis or are feeling overwhelmed by the implications of the choices they must make, yet are feeling an intense need to reach a decision, we encourage them to take a pragmatic approach to problem solving. A pragmatic approach focuses on identifying and considering the concrete factors that will influence each issue. By definition, pragmatic ideas and solutions are easy to understand and clearly applicable to specific circumstances. Therefore we can define a pragmatic approach to problem solving as one that gives clients a tangible means for exploring their options, defines the practical aspects of each issue, and offers realistic solutions to the clients' problems. The following case demonstrates the use of a pragmatic approach to problem solving. David described his dilemma with Jan:

> Jan and I had been using birth control for seven years when we decided we were ready to have kids. We tried for about a year, and then Jan's obstetrician referred us to an infertility specialist. We took sev-

eral tests, and the end result was that Jan would need surgery to correct some problems with her tubes, if we were going to get pregnant.

I can't tell you how disappointed we were. We had already talked about what we could afford to do, and we knew we would have to choose between medical treatment and trying to adopt a baby. We had the money to do one or the other. I felt so cheated. I couldn't believe that it was all coming down to money. We wouldn't even have to consider money if we could get pregnant on our own. Now we had to choose between trying a medical procedure that was a 50–50 chance and trying to adopt. I want to try for adoption and Jan wants to try the surgery, and we can't make a decision between the two with each of us feeling so differently about what is best. The infertility diagnosis is bad enough, but now we are fighting with each other and not making any progress. This whole experience has been a nightmare for us.

EXPLORING OPTIONS.   Jan and David's inability to reach a decision about which option was right for them was based on differing perspectives about the most effective use of their financial resources. Jan had also expressed some discomfort with pursuing adoption before she and David had exhausted all medical options that might allow them to have a biological child, and David had expressed his discomfort with Jan undergoing a surgical procedure, taking the medical risks associated with that procedure, and pursuing biological parenting, when he felt that adoptive parenting was just as desirable. In their efforts to convince one another of the wisdom behind their individual perspectives on this issue, Jan and David had lost sight of the inherent shortcomings of making a decision to bring a child into their lives through a process (a surgical procedure or an adoption) with which one of them was uncomfortable.

It was our impression that Jan and David were both trying to force each other into changing his or her perspective. In doing this, each of them was becoming more and more entrenched in his or her position and less and less able to listen to the other's perspective. To work on this issue we asked Jan and David to complete a decision-making skills inventory (Chapter Eleven). We gave this assignment to Jan and David because it is designed to help clients access their pragmatic problem-solving skills, and it offers a format for making future decisions. We hoped that it would give them some perspective on how to resolve their disagreements about the appropriate path to parenthood. We also wanted them to think about their usual process for making life-altering decisions and to compare that process to the one they had been using to make decisions about parenting.

After completing this exercise Jan and David realized that they were unable to agree on the advantages and disadvantages of each of their options. They did determine that the desired outcome for both of them was parenting. They also determined that in the past they had successfully used lists of pros and cons to make most of their decisions, but when they tried to develop a list of the pros and cons on their alternatives for parenting they could not come up with one that both of them could agree on. They therefore decided that the best option for them was to end treatment until they could decide on an option for parenting with which they both felt comfortable and that they could afford.

Providing Relevant Resources

This skill category relates to the therapeutic process in two distinct ways. First, we must gather information and assess the individual client's existing resources—those that the client is already using or that are readily available to the client (for example, knowledgeable friends or family members, insurance benefits, membership in support groups, or a history of successful problem solving). Second, and most relevant to this discussion, we must maintain current community resource information for our clients.

DEVELOPING A CATALOGUE OF RESOURCES.   You can begin to assemble a resource file by collecting community resource lists, developing an informational brochure, or putting together information packets with brochures and lists that include contact information for resources relevant to your clients' needs. At the very least, you should maintain current resource information about every topic, such as infertility, that you claim as a specialty. For clients who are experiencing infertility, however, you can be of the most help if you are familiar with community resources that offer support and guidance to clients who are undergoing medical treatment, considering adoption or child-free living, or re-experiencing infertility issues in conjunction with other life changes.

We maintain the following resources in our office; you may find them useful in your work with clients who are experiencing infertility. For more information on book and movie titles and on specific organizations, please see Appendixes A and B, respectively.

- Brochures for support groups on infertility, adoption, and child-free living
- Newsletters from organizations that focus on infertility, adoption, surrogacy, parenting, and so on
- Books on adoption, grief and loss, adoption searches and reunions, reproduction, and infertility (covering all aspects of these topics and ranging from titles on openness in adoption to the physical stages of pregnancy and fetal development)
- Articles from journals, magazines, and newspapers; workshop handouts; and information packets that include articles on topics ranging from the home study process and the factors to consider before pursuing an international adoption to brochures exploring medical options for biological parenting
- Flyers from booksellers that specialize in infertility, adoption, and parenting titles
- Community resource directories (Although these resources are usually not specific to clients experiencing infertility, they do offer information on specific organizations that clients may find useful, such as support groups for bereaved parents and hotlines for information on maternal and infant care.)
- Children's books on grief and loss, adoption, coping with developmental changes, and dealing with the addition of a sibling to the family
- Books and movies that do not directly address infertility but that are related to effective coping, decision making, grief, relationships, sexuality, sexual trauma, self-esteem, recovery from addictions, and empowerment

Maintaining community and national resource information will assist you in taking a holistic approach to healing. For instance, if you have a client who is considering adoption and could benefit from individual therapy and participation in a support group, you will be able to guide your client toward an organization that offers a support group for potential adoptive parents. Being familiar with relevant resources entails keeping current information on the quality and type of services provided, fee structures, the population served, service locations, and how to contact the resource. Community resource manuals often contain some of this information, and infertility-related organizations, such as RESOLVE, have helpline volunteers who can answer specific questions.

After receiving a diagnosis of infertility, your clients may need to work with medical specialists, financial planners, attorneys, adoption agencies, support groups, and insurance companies. The constant developments in medical procedures, the particular needs of each client, and the ever-changing alternatives to biological parenting make it impossible for us to do our own research on every issue that confronts our clients. So, in response to our belief that it is critical to update our knowledge base, recycle outdated materials, and share any new or relevant information with our clients, we have found it helpful to join such organizations as Adoptive Families of America (see Appendix B). This organization publishes an extremely informative magazine, which keeps us up-to-date on many of the issues our clients are dealing with. The information is manageable, helpful, and timely, and can easily be passed on to our clients.

MAKING SPECIFIC REFERRALS.   When our clients ask us for a specific referral to an adoption agency, an attorney, or the like, we explain that our policy is not to endorse specific resources but to offer information and references on resources that other clients have found useful. We regularly refer current clients to former clients who have agreed to share their experiences and serve as sources of information about their experiences with various community resources. We offer new clients the option of having direct contact with another client who has been through a similar process, or refer them to a support group that deals with issues similar to those they are dealing with. For instance, when clients are trying to decide whether or not to pursue surrogate parenting, we refer them to a couple who is parenting through surrogacy or to an organization that educates clients about surrogacy, or both. If we know of a particular resource that appears to match the needs of a client, but we have not had experience with the resource, we will locate an individual, agency, resource manual, or helpline that has.

Our policy of nonendorsement is consistent with our general philosophy regarding the tenets of client-therapist relationships: the policy fosters client empowerment. Clients select their own resources and initiate a direct link to the resources they choose. This direct link not only separates us from the resource but also separates us from clients' experiences with the resource. Otherwise we could and would be held responsible for the actions and ethics of independent professionals. It is important to note, however, that we are obligated to warn clients about resources that we have just cause to believe may be harmful to them.

PROVIDING INFORMATION ON ALTERNATIVES TO BIOLOGICAL PARENTING. When you are working in the field of infertility counseling, you must be prepared to discuss alternatives to biological parenting. For this discussion you will need basic information about adoption, surrogacy, donor egg and sperm procedures, and child-free living. You should be familiar with resources that can assist your clients in choosing and pursuing any of these options. You also need to be aware of the specific challenges that each of these options presents. For instance, if a couple is considering surrogate parenting they may need to (1) research local laws on surrogacy, (2) discuss the significance of parenting a child who will be the biological child of one but not the other partner, and (3) weigh the legal and emotional risks of surrogate parenting. You should not be the only person clients consult in making their decisions, because your expertise will naturally be limited to your own discipline and experience. However, you can still be of great use to your clients by providing them with direction, questions for consideration, and referrals to legal and other experts, as well as by helping them assess their suitability for each option. (Chapter Seven and Appendix C describe specific alternatives and detail many of the issues your clients may want to consider before choosing an alternative to biological parenting.)

Although our having a good command of communication and guiding skills is useful in counseling all clients, these skills are *essential* to counseling clients who are experiencing infertility. What makes these skills so relevant relates to the unique impact infertility has on our clients. In the next chapter, we explore that impact.

Understanding the Client Experience with Infertility

〰 Whatever the gains, whatever the losses, they are yours.
—Native American saying

Part Two includes Chapter Three, "Recognizing the Impact of Infertility," and Chapter Four, "Identifying Specific Responses to Infertility." These chapters identify the fundamental issues with which many clients struggle and the range of responses clients may have to their infertility diagnosis. Chapter Three shows how infertility can engender a sense of loss and why an infertility diagnosis can prompt clients to question their gender identity. Chapter Four discusses the gender-specific responses that males and females may have to an infertility diagnosis and responses that relate to which partner receives the diagnosis. It also describes common dilemmas clients face and how infertility can be experienced as a life crisis. These chapters include case examples and strategies for using the exercises provided in Chapter Eleven. Several of the cases introduced here are revisited in the sessions discussed in Chapter Ten.

CHAPTER THREE

Recognizing the Impact of Infertility

Sometime in your life you will go on a journey.
It will be the longest journey you have ever taken.
It is the journey to find yourself.

—*Katherine Sharp, in* Simple Abundance

A client once referred to infertility as "the thief of dreams." He went on to say that infertility robbed him of practically everything he had. This accusation perfectly illustrates the powerlessness and violation clients experience as a result of losing their fertility.

In describing these losses and concerns, clients tell us that infertility changes their entire lives. This chapter explores how an infertility diagnosis can result in a sense of widespread loss, raise questions about gender identity, and challenge the foundation of the couple's relationship.

A SENSE OF WIDESPREAD LOSS

With the loss of fertility comes a host of other losses including the loss of social outlets, sexual well-being, physical comfort, privacy, financial resources, psychological stability, and family harmony. (Specific reproductive losses will be discussed in Chapter Five.)

Isolation

Most couples report a gradual shift in their ability to relate to people with whom they had once talked easily. They notice that it is hard to listen to others because they are forever anticipating the dreaded questions about children: What are their plans and intentions? They are perceived as preoccupied and anxious by their friends, relatives, and coworkers. Some clients eventually withdraw from social settings in an attempt to avoid having to answer awkward questions and listening to the news of others' pregnancies and their children's developmental milestones. With glassy eyes, Nancy says, "If one more person at work gets pregnant that will be the end of me. I just cannot stand it. Why everyone but me and Jason are having kids does not make sense to me. I cannot believe how nosy some people are, too, because they will just come right out and ask us when we are going to have kids. Can you believe it? I do not need to be around all that anyway."

Clients who feel the way Nancy does often choose to rely solely on their partners for what they once acquired from a broad range of individuals. Husbands and wives report increasing frustration with each other and with themselves as they discover the impossibility of meeting all the needs of their spouses. They become unable to do anything out of pure enjoyment because they are always reminded of their isolation and of the fact that there is no one else with whom they can comfortably be.

Although they have isolated themselves, couples may also feel abandoned by their friends and family members who are fearful of saying the wrong thing. And although they are comforted by sharing their pain with each other, they also report feeling resentful that there is no one else with whom they can share the depth of their sadness.

Sexual Problems

The deep sadness that some clients experience permeates every arena of their lives, most notably in their sexual relationship. Some couples no longer feel spontaneous and carefree in their lovemaking because it is so closely associated with their desperate attempt to conceive. Roger says, "How can I approach Julie anymore? The second the spirit moves me I quickly ask myself, 'What night is this? Did we do it last night? Are we allowed to do it again?' By the time I get it all figured out I do not even want to do it. I cannot keep it all straight in my head, and I do not want to be thinking about it anyway. I just want to be doing it."

Many clients report a diminished sex drive due to the need to schedule sex, the loss of spontaneity, and the focus on conception. Couples report that it is impossible to ignore the connection between the physiological function of intercourse with their personal inability to procreate. They find it difficult to have sex for the sheer sake of experiencing pleasure or expressing love. Roger's frustration is understandable and typical for clients who believe that their sexuality is better expressed than examined.

Even after couples decide to discontinue infertility treatment in order to resume more "normal" behaviors, clients express frustration with the seeming presence of infertility in their bedrooms. Once a comfortable expression of their feelings for one another, sexual encounters become laced with sadness for many clients. Dean says, "I just wish we could go back to the way it used to be. I was sure we were going to be fine once we stopped all the injections and planned times for sex. And it is not just Rachel who is crying still. I cannot seem to shake it myself. I have to believe that time is going to fix this. Otherwise, we may as well go back to trying to have a kid so our sadness has some kind of reason for being there." In Chapter Six we discuss ways in which couples in general, and Dean and Rachel specifically, can resume normal sexual functioning and intimacy.

Physical Discomfort

As couples make every attempt to achieve a pregnancy and carry it to full term, they endure a battery of medical examinations and testing procedures. Men and women can experience exams and the numerous physically invasive procedures as uncomfortable and painful. Hormones and medications also can alter a client's usual way of feeling. A woman, particularly, can experience irritability, sluggishness, weight gain, and fatigue. She can also experience pain from daily injections, severe cramping, and side effects induced by the many medications she might be taking. She may experience physical symptoms of her menstrual cycle on a daily basis. Janine said:

I used to be embarrassed by all the talk of PMS and the women who complained about their periods. I could not imagine how someone could be so aware of their body that they knew exactly what day of their cycle they were on. Boy, was I out in left field. This knowing every ache and sign of what is happening inside me is hell. I know that before I just did not have symptoms that I could feel. Now that I do have unpleasant symptoms to contend with, I wish I could say "sorry" to every woman I ever rolled my eyes at.

A Loss of Privacy

Whereas menstrual cycles and frequency of intercourse were once a woman and her partner's private concern, after a diagnosis of infertility a client's cycles and sexual practices are often scrutinized by a number of individuals, from fertility specialists to family members. She is asked specific questions regarding her menstrual and sexual history, former birth control methods, and her general gynecological health. Clara says, "I should just stand on the street corner and shout for everyone to come see the infertile specimen. I may as well. I never thought that so many people would be wandering around down there, poking for this and that while I am supposed to carry on like nothing is going on. Is it really worth all this? I feel like an experiment under a microscope. Do they not see that I am still me?"

The new assisted reproductive technologies often involve an army of medical professionals who monitor sperm counts, egg counts, and body temperatures, as well as ask clients the same intimate questions over and over again. Thus, a couple's sex life becomes a subject of matter-of-fact discussion. They are asked when, how, how often they "do it." They are then advised of the best times to have sex, the best positions to have it in, and how often they should be having sex. Most clients are not prepared to discuss their sexual activities without reservation.

Clients also report that friends and family members provide unsolicited advice about how they should be having sex. Larry told us, "My cousin actually had the nerve to say that I am just not doing it right. He laughed and told me to stop by his place if I wanted to see how it is *really* done. I swear, I should have decked him right there. Did he think I was going to check him and his girl out in the act? Geez."

The comment made by Larry's cousin is well beyond the bounds of propriety, yet we have heard numerous remarks just like it. Most of our clients have repeatedly been asked questions about their intentions to have children and why it is taking them so long to start their family. Many people assume that when a couple does not have children, the couple is willing to discuss their fertility problems openly. (This assumption is similar to the one that leads people to think that a visibly pregnant woman welcomes the feel of a strange hand on her protruding abdomen.) Our clients tell us that all they really want to share with people is the good news of a pregnancy in its second trimester. Clients report that they do not want the matters of their intimate functioning to be the subjects of a public forum. Nor do they wish to discuss the details and expense of their fertility treatment.

Financial Drain

Fertility treatment is expensive. Some procedures alone can cost $10,000 or more per attempt at conception. Most medical health insurance plans place a rigid cap on what they will cover, and a handful will cover nothing at all. Some clients report "losing their shirts" in their attempts to get pregnant. Other clients have facetiously said that the costs of infertility treatment would leave them unable to support a child should they actually get pregnant. Unless a client has an unlimited source of income, money will often determine when clients choose to stop treatment before carrying a successful pregnancy to term.

The drain on clients' financial resources also limits their access to the reproductive technologies that they may be able to participate in, and contributes to their growing sense of powerlessness. In addition, exorbitant costs directly affect the choices clients can make regarding other paths to parenting, such as adoption. Some clients tell us during their adoption consultations that the choice to adopt creates a shift in their hopefulness because "at least now we are not throwing good money after bad." Although clients may feel financially drained by the cost of an adoption, they feel relatively certain that they will ultimately have a child.

In Chapter Seven we discuss how you can help your clients look realistically at their financial situation and determine their subsequent course of action. This will increase your clients' sense that they have the power to effect change in their lives.

Psychological Instability

The single most detrimental effect on clients' psychological functioning is their perceived loss of control throughout infertility treatment. Clients report that their lives become a symbol of their dysfunction because all their behaviors are dramatically affected by their infertility. Janice told us:

> The second I am up in the morning the thermometer is in my mouth, and I lay like a corpse fearful that the slightest movement, even a breath, will affect the temperature reading. Of course, from there my mood goes up or down with the reading. My life revolves around scheduled appointments to have sex, scheduled appointments with specialists, and contrived scheduled events designed to avoid bumping into anyone who might be happy. Just the simple question "How are you?" makes my emotions well up with an intensity that scares me. I am exhausted. Everyday I face myself in the mirror and wonder how my life got so hard to deal with. I wonder, too, how long I can keep up the facade that everything is fine, even though my life feels so empty. I hate my obsession to get pregnant and yet it is genuinely all I care about. And I hate to think of what my husband thinks of the mess he is married to. I just have no idea what to do with myself.

Janice possessed the self-awareness to see how she had allowed infertility to consume her life, but she also expressed that she was unable to help herself untangle "the mess" she had become. Like all obsessions, the obsession to get pregnant becomes the lens through which the client sees the world. Individuals experiencing infertility view every woman on the street and every woman in their social and familial circles as pregnant or as having small children. They may be particularly in tune to crying babies and the absence of an immediately comforting parent. They may feel as though they are nothing if they are not a father or a mother. The obsession to become parents causes clients to lose touch with their true identity, and renders them unable to make life choices and manage their behaviors appropriately.

Family Discord

Many couples report that infertility replaces family harmony with discord. Because each individual responds uniquely to his or her predicament, it can become increasingly difficult for partners to understand each other or express themselves clearly. The sense of despair about the infertility and the feelings of not being understood by the partner can result in poor communication between couples. A breakdown in communication inevitably results in tension between partners, and in subsequent arguments, withdrawal from each other, or both. By the time clients initiate therapy, individual partners may present as disconnected from each other as they live in their own private misery. The downward spiral from family harmony toward family discord seems to be a direct result of the different ways in which men and women translate the meaning of the infertility into their individual self-concepts.

QUESTIONS ABOUT GENDER IDENTITY

We express our *learned* ideas about gender and what it means to be masculine and feminine through our style of dress, our mannerisms, our sexuality and sexual relationships, and sometimes in our choice of professions (although gender is becoming a less significant factor in this arena). Perhaps the most *inherent* ideas we have about gender are based on our biological roles in reproduction.

Infertility has an impact on our clients' abilities to fulfill their gender-specific, biological roles in the reproductive process. Women assume that they can get pregnant. Men assume they can impregnate. They both assume that the choice is theirs. Infertility defies these basic assumptions about what it means to be female or male and seemingly robs clients of their reproductive choices. In this culture, procreation is viewed as an entitlement, and the "inability" to reproduce is viewed as a fundamental deficiency. The impact of infertility on each gender varies according to roles that men and women play in reproduction, but there is a common link: both genders experience losses as the result of an infertility diagnosis. (For a woman it may be the loss of physically carrying the child in her womb, and for a man it may be the loss of being the support person throughout the pregnancy.) Therefore, effective infertility counseling must address the general loss of the ability to reproduce (which we explore in Chapter Five), the formation of gender identity, and how infertility affects masculinity and femininity.

Gender Identity

In order to understand fully why infertility can have such a profound impact on our clients' identities as men and women, we must first understand the influence that gender has on identity formation. Cultural distinctions are made between boys and girls from the moment of birth. Parents, relatives, peers, television, books, advertising, and religious doctrine impart values about gender to children. Children who express themselves in gender-inappropriate ways are singled out, chastised, and sometimes humiliated for not conforming to gender standards. In *Bastard out of Carolina,* for example, Dorothy Allison describes the games that the heroine, Bone, and her female cousins and friends play when they tire of playing with the boys:

> "We're gonna play mean sisters."
> "What?"
> "We're gonna play mean sisters," I told them all again, . . . "[F]irst we're gonna play Johnny Yuma's mean sisters, then Francis Marion's mean sisters, then Bat Masterson's. Then we'll think of somebody else."
> Reese looked confused. "What do mean sisters do?"
> "They do everything their brothers do. Only they do it first and fastest and meanest."
> "Yeah! I want to be the Rifleman's mean sister."

Allison goes on to describe how the heroine's family members overhear the girls' game and think their children have gone crazy. When confronted by their bewildered elders, one "mean sister," Patsy Ruth, is humiliated by her participation in the game and immediately blames Bone for making up the game in the first place. She does this even though they were all apparently empowered by and thoroughly engrossed in their new pastime. Sadly, Patsy Ruth's reaction is quite typical in this situation. Nonconformity to gender-specific expectations is a dire sin, indeed.

Infertility sometimes prevents men and women from conforming to (or, more accurately, from meeting) the reproductive expectations that are placed on them, both as human beings and as males and females. The meaning that infertility will take on in clients' lives will vary by gender. These differences are expected, because the roles in reproduction are often gender defined. When an infertility diagnosis assaults our clients' gender identity, some of the losses they experience are also related to their gender. When we understand the impact of infertility on gender identity, we are better able to understand the losses our clients are experiencing.

A significant part of gender education relates to the male and female roles in the reproductive process. Therefore, our clients' infertility diagnosis undermines their self-concept or identity as a male or female. We look first at how men's gender identity can be affected by infertility, and then at how women's gender identity can be affected.

How Infertility Affects Masculinity

Although exceptions to gender-specific rules are thankfully becoming more common, most people still have definite values about what is appropriate for each gender. As we said earlier, parents impart their expectations for their sons from the moment they learn of their child's gender. Boys who cry are sissies; boys can go outside without their shirts on; boys learn to problem-solve through aggression and reason; boys grow up to be daddies.

Men who are (or whose partners are) diagnosed with infertility are faced with a potential assault on their manhood. Because masculinity is associated with virility, potency, and strength, infertility is conversely associated with impotency, weakness, and being effeminate. A man who cannot reproduce is simply unmanly. These cultural standards of what it means to be male and masculine are an intrinsic part of the male child's socialization. These are the standards by which the male child judges his "fit" into his own gender and by which he is judged by others, both male and female.

So how do these cultural standards of manhood affect the identity of the male client who is experiencing infertility? Our male clients report that infertility causes them to feel as though the legitimacy of their identity as a man, a husband, and a potential father is being challenged, both by society and by the man himself.

Of course, the degree to which men identify with this view of masculinity varies from person to person. Furthermore, not all men experience infertility this way, but for those who do or who have friends or family who affiliate masculinity with procreation, infertility strikes at the very core of their male identity. The individual man may not perceive himself as less masculine, but most of our clients can name at least one other person in their life whom they believe sees them as less masculine. In our experience, men who do not suffer from some aspect of this view of masculinity and infertility are rare.

How Infertility Affects Femininity

Parents impart their expectations for their daughters from the moment they learn of their child's gender. Girls learn to problem-solve through persuasion and discussion; girls learn to cross their legs in order to be "ladylike"; girls who prefer more masculine activities are "tomboys"; girls grow up to be mommies.

Infertility presents women with a complex variety of challenges and emotions, which by nature of her gender and socialization she feels obligated to unravel. One such reaction is the response that some women have to the loss of the experience of pregnancy and childbirth. This loss can be experienced as both a physical and psychological assault on the woman's identity. From the physical perspective, pregnancy and childbirth are normal functions of a woman's body and are universally understood. Furthermore, the decision for a woman to procreate or not is often understood to depend on prerogative as opposed to limitation. In the biological sense, the female body is in a continuous state of preparation for pregnancy, through the monthly cycles of menstruation (which last for approximately thirty years of the woman's life). Women are thus reminded on a monthly basis of their biological role in procreation.

The biological expectation that all females are potential mothers is coupled with a cultural expectation that all females desire motherhood. Little girls are given dolls to practice on through play, and are encouraged to exhibit characteristics that lend themselves to "good mothering." For example, little girls are "good little girls" when they are nurturing, loving, feminine, and caring. Many of the toys for girls are related to the roles of wife and mother, such as doll houses, miniature household appliances, and various other toys that relate to taking care of others (shopping carts, animals that require grooming and dressing, and dolls that need their diapers changed). As young women and adults, females are further prepared for motherhood through television programs, advertising, home economics courses, and babysitting. The underlying message is that motherhood is the ultimate expression of femininity.

What does this message mean for the woman whose body is not capable of pregnancy? And what is the impact of the monthly reminder of the lost potential for motherhood? For many of our female clients, these two questions are at the core of their doubts about their identity as women. Women begin to ask themselves who they can be if they cannot be a mother. It is as if their human value has been reduced, and their whole being, body and soul, has become "infertile." Infertility is no longer a medical condition but a definition of self.

For one client, Maria, her grief over the loss of the pregnancy experience had become incapacitating. Maria was no longer able to see herself as anything other than an "infertile woman." She had lost perspective on her value as a person and on the other roles she played in her life that contributed to her identity: wife, gardener, sister, daughter, and homemaker. Maria presented the following description of her current state of mind during our initial session:

> The other day my husband asked me if I was going to let the weeds take over the garden. I told him, and I know this sounds stupid, that I could not believe that he was pointing out my failure to take care of flowers, when he knew very well that I felt bad enough about my failure to grow a baby. It sounds crazy, but I guess I think that I cannot make anything grow anymore. I know that the garden has nothing to do with the infertility, but for me I just cannot face all of that work to get the garden to grow, so that I can watch it die. It is just too much.
>
> All I know is that if I was going to be a mother, I would feel like my life was complete. But since I am not, I guess I better figure out what I am going to do with the rest of my life. I just cannot imagine ever feeling good about anything again. I do not even know if my husband will stay with me when he realizes that children are not an option for us. My guess is that he will find someone who will be able to give him a baby. Since I cannot do that, I cannot imagine that he would be happy with me. I am not happy with me.

Maria's self-described obsession with getting pregnant had become the primary focus of her life. She had become so despondent over the loss of motherhood that she also lost her capacity to find any joy in the other roles that she played in her life. Although this example may seem like an extreme, it is not. It is true, however, that some of Maria's emotions were more intense than those of other clients, and not everyone is this depressed after medical intervention fails. Nonetheless, the themes in Maria's story (questioning her value as a wife, feeling that the inability to get pregnant has lowered her value as a woman, and believing that she is incapable of nurturing anything, because she cannot "grow a baby") are typical for many women who have allowed infertility to sabotage their self-concepts.

As we have discussed, gender strongly influences the individual client's response to infertility and its losses. The influence of gender is due to socialization, to a tendency to define life and its circumstances in terms of opposites (good-bad, male-female, fruitful-barren, creative-unproductive, emotional-logical), to biological functions, and to personal beliefs about what makes people valuable.

The therapeutic process should begin with untangling the infertility from the client's identity. It is important for both partners to be a part of the therapy, because each person will bring a different perspective into the process, and each perspective will have an impact on the relationship. Infertility is certainly a part of your client's gender identity, but it does not define it. Your task will be to help them see that.

IMPACT ON THE RELATIONSHIP

For men whose female partners are the identified medical patient, overcompensation, when it occurs, is chiefly apparent in the man's attempts to make their partners feel better. Men, at least in this culture, are vigorously socialized to "fix" problems. Their genuine desire to be supportive and useful is often misconstrued by their female partner as a lack of empathy. Misunderstandings happen because the man is not expressing emotions similar to those of his female partner. Whereas the man is trying to fix the problem (the infertility and his partner's distress), the woman is trying to engage him in her process of comprehending and expressing both partners' feelings about the infertility. It is not surprising, then, that partners can become alienated from each other. The next two sections explore gender-specific responses to infertility and the all too common belief that a pregnancy will solve marital problems.

Gender-Specific Responses

The following case illustrates the common effects of infertility on a male-female couple and their relationship. Jason recalls his and Nancy's experience after they experienced a miscarriage:

> We were both so stuck in trying to get the other person to see our point of view that we stopped listening to each other. Nancy felt like I thought she was going off the deep end . . . and I guess in some ways I did. I kept trying to pull her back from the edge by telling her that the only way we were going to get through this was by figuring out each decision as it came up. I just did not see how worrying about what was going to happen was going to get us anywhere.
>
> Now, I think that she was just trying to tell me that she was scared and I just could not think about every possibility without going nuts. The more I tried to get her to calm down and take it one step at a time,

the more she accused me of not really caring about whether or not we ever had a baby. I know she thought that I was not as attached to the baby as she was. It is not that I did not care. I was really upset about the whole infertility thing and I was really excited when we found out we were pregnant. I just did not see how being upset all the time was going to change anything. It seemed like we had painted ourselves into opposite corners of a room and all we could do was point out how the other person was responsible.

In this situation, Jason and Nancy are behaving in typically male and female ways. For example, Jason's attempts at damage control through problem solving requires skills that men are expected to learn and use in a crisis. Women, on the other hand, are encouraged to express their feelings, as Nancy did, and to manage the emotional aspects of a crisis. However, the differences between the roles that males and females are expected to play in crisis management have, in this situation, led Nancy to believe that Jason was not feeling the loss of their child. When these kinds of misunderstandings remain unresolved, women may find themselves grieving not only the losses of infertility but also the potential loss of their emotional relationship with their partner. Men wind up feeling misunderstood and inadequate in their attempts to solve the problem.

To help Nancy and Jason restore a sense of balance in the relationship, we knew we would have to guide each of them from their extreme end of the spectrum toward the middle: Jason needed to be able to experience his grief through the expression of his feelings, and Nancy needed to identify and discuss the couple's options through problem solving. This shifting of roles allows each partner to deepen his or her understanding of and appreciation for the value of the other partner's coping skills. We gave Jason and Nancy a homework assignment to facilitate the process of restoring balance to their relationship. We explained the assignment in the following way:

> We would like you to have a very structured conversation, with rules and everything. Each one of you will have fifteen minutes to explain to the other one what your point of view is about anything that you feel is a problem. During each person's fifteen minutes, the other person is not supposed to do anything but listen, and ask questions if they do not understand something. Then it is the next person's turn. Even though you may find it difficult not to interject your opinion, or to

clarify a point, you need to remain silent, except for questions, for the full fifteen minutes.

Jason and Nancy did their homework, and Nancy gave the following description of their experience:

> It was really hard not to correct him when he talked about things I did not agree with, and I know he had a hard time with it too. I used all of my questions to ask Jason how he felt about whatever he was talking about, and he was really good about trying to answer me. Whenever I would say things like, "I just do not know what to do," he would ask me if I was able to think of anything that might make me feel better. It is kind of funny: we both stuck to our emotion and logic thing, but it was different because we were asking instead of telling. Some of his questions actually helped me to see some of my choices, and I know it was a relief for him to talk about how sad he was about the miscarriage.
>
> I think that having rules really helped Jason, and for the first time in a long time, I really felt like he was listening to me instead of trying to tell me why I should not let something upset me. After we began to have to listen to each other, it started to get easier to see the other person's point of view. It is a strange way to talk to someone you have known for eight years, but it really seemed to help us.

Many of the couples we work with present gender-specific issues. For instance, men often express feelings of responsibility to continue the family line; these feelings are based on expectations that are traditionally imposed on men. Women often tell us that they believe their male partners see their grief reaction as "irrational and too emotional" and describe their male partners as "too unfeeling and logical." Clearly, these characteristics are identified as typically *female* or *male* in nature.

In any event, we strive to let clients know that their reactions are not right or wrong. Rather, what needs to be examined is whether or not their reactions to the diagnosis and to each other are contributing to a sense of isolation from one another. If the answer is yes, the isolation may very well be a result of clients' relying on gender stereotypes to interpret and then judge the prudence of their own behavior and that of their partner. Although gender clearly has an influence on our clients' reactions to an infertility diagnosis, that the reaction is gender-specific does not mean that it is an invalid or unworthy response. When we or our clients place an individual's reaction into an oversimplified gender category, we run the risk of limiting our ability to listen to and accept our client's perspective.

Although we have outlined the most prevalent influences that gender will have on clients who are experiencing infertility, we also recognize that there are always exceptions to the rules. We learn a tremendous amount from working with clients who respond to an infertility diagnosis in an atypically gender-neutral fashion, because these clients who don't "follow" gender-based rules or who defy the usual standards of behavior may also be coping in an extremely effective manner. They can teach us about dislodging the obstacles of gender stereotypes from individual relationships.

Couples may continue to feel alienated from each other even after gender stereotypes are exposed and dismantled. Continued feelings of alienation seem to result when clients are unable to derive meaning from their suffering, regardless of their efforts to do so. We have found that some couples cannot untangle their nonproductive behaviors and find peace in the practical or philosophical answers they have obtained, nor can they accept that some of their questions will remain unanswered. Couples who fall into this category risk experiencing further difficulty with perception and functioning inside their relationship. We have seen this difficulty evidenced in couples' beliefs that a pregnancy will solve the problems in the (marital) relationship.

Belief That a Pregnancy Will Solve Marital Problems

It is normal for fulfilled, stable couples to spend a lot of time and energy attending to the pursuit of biological parenting. But stable couples do not allow their experience with infertility to override the importance of the other interests and endeavors they share with one another. Clients who are not fulfilled in their marriages often hope that a pregnancy will create increased contentment in the marriage. Some clients instinctively justify their obsession with biological parenting with the belief that a pregnancy will solve the marital problems that existed prior to the infertility diagnosis. Essentially, when conception is problematic, it only delays the emergence of the core problems in the partnership. Similarly, when a couple achieves a healthy pregnancy, they will be only temporarily distracted from their previous conflicts.

Couples who believe that a pregnancy will solve marital problems risk further deterioration of the marriage. We have seen two distinct consequences to this belief: (1) the marriage becomes a relationship based solely on infertility and the dream of biological parenting, or (2) children either born to, or subsequently adopted into, this union become the focus of the marriage, with subsequent inappropriate expectations placed on them.

MARRIAGE BASED ON INFERTILITY.   When the marriage becomes a relationship based solely on infertility and the dream of biological parenting, the marriage is at risk for deterioration. Clients who, prior to their diagnosis, were already experiencing difficulty with communication, shared goals, or common value systems may see their experience with infertility as an opportunity to align with each other for a cause. Thus the infertility gives new meaning to the marriage. On the surface, this view appears to possess the promise of rediscovery or reconnection between marriage partners. Underlying the promise, however, are the original unresolved problems, which will inevitably resurface. The couple will then find themselves unable to navigate the infertility experience, just as they have been unable to navigate the core problems in the marriage. They discover that it is impossible to conceal or ignore their core problems even if they achieve a pregnancy.

We encourage intensive marital therapy to help these couples build a solid foundation of skills that can guide them through their marital difficulties. You might want to begin your work with this type of couple in a noninvasive manner. We recommend that you ask each partner to work in their journals on the following questions (see Chapter Eleven for a more complete guide to journal writing):

1. List six to eight important events in your life. Be sure to include descriptions as well as feelings.

2. For every path you have chosen in life, another path was not taken. Regarding the aforementioned events, answer the following questions: What choices were not made? What did you actively accept or reject? What would your life be like now if . . . Create a dialogue between your current self and the self that might have emerged had you taken a different path.

3. Consider your options for the future. Is there anything you are currently doing that you would like to alter? What would it take for you to do that? What is the best thing that could happen to you? What is the worst thing that could happen to you? How committed are you to acting on this? What will your plan of

action be? What will you have to give up in order to make this change? Are you willing to venture into new, undiscovered territory? What will support you on your new road?

The answers to these questions will not only come to light for individual clients but will help you see just how connected or disconnected from one another the partners in the couple are. You can use the information as a starting place for augmenting the dreams they share, in order to rebuild the roads that have crumbled between them. Without therapeutic intervention, clients may completely lose touch with the qualities and reasons that initially drew them together. They may experience increased conflict with or withdrawal from each other, and without intervention, the foundation of the marriage inevitably crumbles.

CHILD-FOCUSED MARRIAGES.   Children either born to or adopted into these unions become the focus of the marriage and subsequently have inappropriate expectations placed on them. Parents who focus all their attention on the children they so desperately struggled to acquire may unwittingly believe that their children's presence will be a panacea for the difficulties in the marriage. This belief cannot be further from the truth. Instead, the presence of children in unstable relationships only *emphasizes* and complicates the problems in the marriage.

Initially, when the child is young and nonverbal, it may seem to the parents that everything is fine. Their longed-for baby has arrived, and the baby's needs are relatively easy to meet because they are primarily physical. A parent may eventually feel as though they have no use for their problematic marriage now that they have what appears to be a loving parent-child relationship.

As children get older and are more capable of meeting their own physical needs, their psychological and emotional needs increase and the demands on their parents become more complicated. It was easy for the parents to feed a hungry baby, but it is difficult to answer questions about identity development and peer relationships. Thus, the parents struggle to meet the needs of their child that have gone unmet in the marriage, and the strain between partners becomes even greater than it once was. These parents who expected their children to solve their relationship issues have made an unconscious assumption that their children's needs will be secondary to their needs. Additionally, these parents are continually disappointed with their children for not resolving all the parents' problems. Essentially, the children of these unstable marriages are not appreciated as unique individuals in their own right but are seen as objects acquired for the ultimate purpose of solving the problems in their parents' marriage.

Because it is impossible for children to solve their parents' problems, eventually *all* of the family dynamics become dysfunctional. Couples may then wonder what happened to their dream of parenting. Parents question the meaning of their past decisions and subsequently blame their children for their disenchantment. These parents do not realize that they, not their children, are responsible for the deterioration of the dream.

When a couple appears to rely on a pregnancy to solve their marital problems, we recommend that medical treatment for the infertility be temporarily postponed. We are very candid about our concerns, and we explain the long-term implications of the couple's beliefs. Many people reject our recommendation and expect to "deal with that issue" if they become pregnant, because they don't wish to stop the clock in their pursuit of biological parenting. Some of those who do accept our recommendation, however, are able to resolve their problems. Some couples choose to part. Ultimately, many of these couples discover new meaning in their lives and new relationships as a result of the therapeutic process. Whether couples remain together or choose to part, we would expect that the prospective children of these individuals will have a better chance of being parented by individuals who can appropriately meet their needs.

Comprehending the impact of infertility on the individual client requires an understanding of the connections between infertility, identity, loss, and gender. An infertility diagnosis changes clients' usual way of functioning and challenges their ability to manifest the cultural definitions of gender. As we have seen, changes in functioning encompass every aspect of clients' personal life. Furthermore, clients who are experiencing infertility also perceive a shift in their ability to meet the cultural standards of their gender and maintain their identities as men and women, husbands and wives. The extent to which a client's overall functioning is impaired after a diagnosis of infertility is directly related to the individual's response to the changes in his or her life. We now move on to discuss specific ways in which men and women respond to the infertility experience.

CHAPTER FOUR

Identifying Specific
Responses to Infertility

*Everywhere man is confronted with fate, with the chance
of achieving something through his own suffering.*

—*Viktor Frankl,* Man's Search for Meaning

Clients' responses to an infertility diagnosis are very complex. Some are directly related to the person's gender; others have more to do with the particular diagnosis; still others have more to do with the reactions other people have to their friend or family member's predicament. Although some clients can endure the diagnosis with very little turmoil, at the other end of the spectrum are clients who respond to the diagnosis of infertility and ensuing treatment as a profound blow to their life's dreams and their self-concept.

In this chapter we examine all of these particular responses that clients may experience after a diagnosis of infertility. Although we explore them separately, it is important to note that they are not mutually exclusive: one client may experience several of these responses at any given point in the infertility ordeal. We begin by continuing our discussion of gender from Chapter Three but shift our focus from the impact of gender on infertility to the responses that are typically male and typically female. We then discuss responses that relate to whether the infertility diagnosis is a result of one or both partners' physiological problems. Next we examine specific dilemmas that many clients face and the possible responses they may have to those dilemmas. Finally, we explore infertility as a life crisis.

MALE RESPONSES

The "standard" of the male as an unemotional being (in contrast to the standard of females as emotional beings) usually results in a mandate for the repression of many of a man's *human* emotions, particularly sadness and despair. However, the expression of anger in its verbal form is almost always acceptable for men. Physical expressions of anger are also acceptable, but less so than verbal expressions. Our culture rationalizes that when men express anger and frustration, they are just being their *naturally aggressive* selves. Therefore, it is not unusual for us to see men in our practice who deal with their grief through expressions of anger.

In theory, grief is understood in part to include anger, but anger does not define the whole of grief. (See Chapter Five for stages of grief.) As men move beyond their anger, they may begin to experience emotions with which they are unfamiliar or uncomfortable. It is at this point that many men fall back on their "training" and use repression as a coping mechanism. Consequently, men often find it difficult to accept openly grieving the losses associated with infertility and to give themselves permission to do so (and by *grieve* we mean fully experience the range of their emotions).

Most frequently, men oversee their grief and manifest their repressed emotions through overcompensation in other areas of their life. They tend to focus their energy on areas in which they feel most competent and that traditionally foster the male's self-esteem: work, athletics, and problem solving. (Problem solving with infertility commonly appears in the form of a logical, step-by-step plan for combating the infertility, reaching the goal of biological parenting, or both.) Thus, this problem-solving response to infertility honors the traditional standard of men as steadfast and unemotional.

The historically male role as the head of the household and protector of family members implies that a man must be strong, fearless, and heroic. The man who has been encouraged to express his "manly and unmanly" emotions and freely does so is often judged as not manly enough, as effeminate. He will most likely be perceived as too emotional to fulfill the obligations of his masculine roles. This judgment will be imposed with or without a diagnosis of infertility. From a therapeutic standpoint, his emotional expressions ought not to be discouraged but instead acknowledged and appreciated. However, if he is feeling unable to strike a balance between his emotional reactions and his composure, it would be appropriate to incorporate his concerns into the treatment plan, as we did with George in Chapter One. As you may recall, George struggled with the definition of his masculinity, and was able to design a ritual that honored his need to problem solve and acknowledged his feelings of loss.

FEMALE RESPONSES

Whereas our male clients may struggle with learning to experience a broader range of emotions, our female clients often struggle with managing the range of emotions they are already experiencing. Women have a tendency to carry the emotional burdens for the members of their family, and this has certainly been a defining characteristic of the female clients we have counseled around the issues of infertility. As noted earlier, men are more likely to seek external control of their environments, whereas women are inclined to seek internal control through an awareness and understanding of the origins of their emotions.

When we work with female clients who are experiencing infertility, we often see them trying to manage the emotional impact of the infertility for both themselves and their partners. For instance, women will attempt to engage their male partners in discussions about their grief and want to know how he is feeling about the infertility experience. Women often report that their male partners are not easily engaged in such conversations, and that their male partner's reluctance to discuss his feelings leaves them with the perception that they are alone in their grief, that their partners are not experiencing the infertility in the same way they are: "He doesn't seem to understand what a tremendous emotional impact this is having on me," and "His reserve makes me feel like a basket case."

When women are feeling alone in their grief, we discuss the differences between male and female coping mechanisms and explain that many of the differences in reactions between men and women are based on socialization. We also strive to validate each gender's and each individual's reaction to an infertility diagnosis, and then try to help our clients see the value in one another's reactions. Although everyone has the potential ability to appreciate the reaction of his or her spouse, there are some reactions that are hard to convey and thus difficult for the partner to understand. One such difficult reaction is the initial response to learning which partner has been diagnosed with infertility.

RESPONSES TO LEARNING WHO HAS BEEN DIAGNOSED WITH INFERTILITY

So far in our discussion of the loss of the imagined biological child, we have assumed that the experience of infertility is shared equally by both partners. Although the experience is shared theoretically, it is normal for individuals to feel relieved when they are not the one who is diagnosed with the problem. Additionally, it is common for diagnosed partners to feel guilty when they are the one who receives the medical diagnosis.

The *individual* partners' response to their shared fate will determine how the *relationship* is affected by an infertility diagnosis. The relationship is therefore likely to experience a degree of turbulence, as most people are not adequately prepared to find themselves in this quandary. The way in which couples deal with infertility presents unique obstacles for the couple to navigate.

Combined Diagnosis

Statistics show that 40 percent of all cases of infertility are due to the combined problems of both partners. A joint medical problem can be frustrating because a solution to one partner's problems is not necessarily a panacea for the infertility. Some couples experience profound despair over the seemingly impossible difficulties they must overcome, whereas others take a matter-of-fact approach to their predicament. Catherine and Bob's pragmatic approach to their shared diagnosis is evidenced in the following letter:

> When we found out that Bob's sperm count was low and had low motility, we were worried because Catherine had already been diagnosed with severely blocked tubes. We wondered how Bob's sperm was ever going to get where it needed to go because it did not have the numbers, the power, or an avenue! We were very fortunate because we responded to IVF after six tries, despite our conditions that were never actually corrected. For us, the process of infertility treatment required

patience for the ever-changing technology and perseverance through each failed attempt.

A medical diagnosis in both partners can alleviate some stress in the relationship because each partner is in a better position to understand the other's personal loss. Because no one person holds the diagnosis alone, both partners can share any guilt and regret they may experience.

In 5 to 10 percent of couples who receive standardized testing, nothing is "wrong" with either partner, and the diagnosis is "unexplained infertility." In rare cases the infertility is a result of the combined chemical or chromosomal makeup of each partner. Some couples experience this predicament as devastating because there is no possibility of producing healthy offspring with one another. In situations like this, we have seen couples choose child-free living, adoption, and surrogacy as alternatives. They usually make these choices after having gained some self-understanding through their work on the homework exercises we provide (Chapter Eleven), such as considering child-free living, decision-making skills inventory, and when to discontinue treatment. Self-discovery facilitates clients' sharing their experience of infertility.

Truly sharing the *experience* implies that partners are able to refrain from blaming and withdrawing from one another, and to support one another without regard for what the individual medical issues are. Although it is possible to genuinely share the infertility experience, most couples do not arrive at this juncture without a struggle. Joint therapy can help enable partners to function in a supportive, nurturing manner. However, it is critical to allow partners to vent their individual frustrations and disappointments *before* attempting to help them see each other's point of view. This venting is usually best handled in separate sessions. Then you can begin to emphasize the importance of each person's ability to manage his or her own response to the diagnosis. Ultimately, your clients should be able to separate the diagnosis from the person who holds the diagnosis.

Using the integrity wheel exercise (Chapter Eleven) can facilitate this process. This tool was developed to help clients see all aspects of their identity in relation to their entire being. It is a blank pie chart that clients fill in with individual statements that represent components of their identity. This exercise is versatile, as it can be adapted to convey the integrity of individuals, relationships, and predicaments.

The integrity wheel is also helpful for clients who are the only one in the partnership to have received a diagnosis of infertility.

Individual Diagnosis

In the remaining 60 percent of all infertility cases, infertility is found equally in men and women. When we cover infertility treatment histories in our first session with a couple, clients tell us, almost at the onset of the session, which partner "checks out" and which one does not. It is typical for men who "check out" to be the ones to let us know that this is the case. We rarely hear a man blame his wife for the problem, but it is obviously important to him that we know he is "fine." It seems important, too, that men demonstrate their unimpaired states even further by appearing to be emotionally supportive of their spouses by being strong throughout the infertility journey. This reaction is understandable in a culture that expects men to remain strong even in the face of sadness, fear, and confusion.

Conversely, when it is the woman who "checks out," she typically is not the one who volunteers this information. We have observed that women feel guilty when they *are* the ones with the medical problem and feel guilty when they are *not* the ones with the problem. It is as though the woman believes she is not "woman enough" to improve her husband's virility, and will remain quiet while her husband delivers their infertility history. Understanding these dynamics between partners will facilitate your helping them separate their responses to the diagnosis itself from their responses to the implications that the diagnosis will have in their lives. As we have said, there are of course clients who do respond differently; they are very matter-of-fact, and view the situation as a shared one regardless of who actually holds the diagnosis.

DILEMMAS

Through our work with clients and through the stories they have told us, we have identified specific dilemmas that often arise for clients who are experiencing infertility. The dilemmas we have identified include how to manage questions and comments from family and friends, how to deal with holidays and family-focused celebrations, how to cope with other people's pregnancies, how to integrate one's own sexual history, and how to accept the parenting practices of others. The next sections explore these dilemmas.

Managing Questions from Family and Friends

Clients frequently report that they struggle to find an appropriate way to answer the infertility-related questions that family and friends ask. Clients describe questions from "well-meaning" others about their specific options and decisions for medical treatment, sexual practices, delayed childbearing, methods of dealing with grief, and the effects of the infertility on the marital or long-term relationship. Aside from struggling with appropriate responses to these questions, clients also struggle to determine who is in fact entitled to an answer.

Regarding whether a response is appropriate and warranted, we begin by giving our clients permission to firmly decline to answer any question they do not want to answer. We do this by validating our client's right to privacy and by using analogies to explore the appropriateness of the questions being asked. For example, we might ask our clients if they believe that it would be appropriate to walk up to an acquaintance and ask her to describe her sexual preferences in terms of position, timing, and desired outcomes. Clearly, most clients, and people in general, would agree that this question is inappropriate.

We also discuss the right to privacy by exploring the relationship between clients' telling family and friends about the infertility diagnosis and the assumption that having this knowledge entitles the recipient to additional information. Regardless of whether it is the client, the friend or family member, or both who are making the assumption about entitlement to more information, they are doing only that: making an assumption. The act of telling someone about the infertility diagnosis does not include an implicit request by the client to be questioned, nor does it entitle those who have been told about the diagnosis to receive answers to further questions.

Once we address the issues of entitlement and appropriate questioning with our clients, we begin to explore the issue of our clients' responses to the questions and comments of family and friends. Our clients tell us that they often hesitate to use responses that they perceive may alienate the person who asked the questions. The following case tells the story of Greg and Gina's experience with this dilemma.

GINA: In the beginning stages of treatment, I welcomed any opportunity to talk about the infertility. But over the last few months, I have really started to resent the questions and the advice that everyone in my family has been giving me. I don't know if the comments have become more personal or if I have just gotten more sensitive. I guess I just don't have any perspective anymore. I do know that my family has been supportive, and I don't know how to tell them how I feel without it seeming like I'm ungrateful.

I have gone from giving people detailed explanations of the treatment process to imagining how good it would feel to respond to personal questions by saying something like, "What makes you think that our sex life is any of your business?" or "You know, I don't remember asking you for your advice." Even though I know I could say things like that, I also know that most people would be really offended and probably don't realize how intrusive some of their questions can be. I guess the bottom line is that I feel like I opened the bedroom door to everyone I told about the infertility, and now I want to go back and close it.

GREG: Just because we told people about the infertility and talked about our feelings doesn't mean that we wanted people to try to solve our problems or to help us to figure out what we might be doing wrong, you know, with our sexual relationship. It's like a free-for-all on Greg and Gina's infertility every time we get together with our families. I'm really sick of it, and I wish that people would realize that there is a difference between being supportive and giving advice.

It's as if they all think that we have spent the last year of our lives living in a dream world and have never considered why this is happening or what we can do about it. Well, if the agony we have gone through is living in a dream world, I'm ready to wake up.

We have both reached a point where we want to put an end to the questions, mostly because we'd like to be around our families without always having to think about the infertility, but we don't know how to tell them to stop asking. We will talk about it, when we want to, just like everybody else who has a problem is allowed to do.

THERAPIST: From what you have said it seems like you are not only struggling with wanting the questions to stop but also with finding a way to let people know how you feel about their questions and comments without alienating anyone. I have noticed during our previous counseling sessions that the two of you are consistently able to use humor to relieve your stress. I have also noticed that each of you has an appreciation for the other's sense of humor. Would you agree with that?

GREG: Yes. I know we laugh all of the time, and Gina's sense of humor is one of the things that attracted me to her in the first place.

GINA: I think it is true, too. We are always laughing our way out of one disagreement or another. In fact, both of us come from families that have their share of comedians. I think it's one of the reasons why we all get along as well as we do.

THERAPIST: Humor just seems to be so much a part of your communication that I was thinking you might be able to use it to deflect some of the questions that are being asked and to respond to comments that are making you uncomfortable. For instance, do you remember the story you told me about that woman in the supermarket?

GINA: Do you mean my friend who trapped me in the deli line and started asking questions about when we were going to have children?

THERAPIST: Yes. I remember your telling me that Greg walked up behind her, and when he realized what the discussion was about, he started acting like he was going to throw some of the stuff in his hands at her. You two were laughing so hard you could barely tell the story.

GREG: Gina almost burst out laughing right in her face. It was really funny to watch her try not to laugh. You know, I think this could work, especially with our families. Even if we just kept the joke between us it might make it easier to get through certain situations.

Because both Greg and Gina agreed that humor was a "natural" for them and that it had always been an effective coping skill, we began to explore ways they could use humor to reduce their stress about questions and comments from others. They believed that this approach would have positive results because most of their family and friends used humor themselves and understood Greg and Gina's tendency to use humor in stressful situations.

We also suggest that clients prepare themselves for future situations where questions are likely to be asked, such as at a family get-together. Clients can work on anticipating events that might pose a problem and try to make decisions about how they might handle these situations. We also discuss the benefits of having prepared answers to questions about children, pregnancy, and parenting. Prepared answers eliminate the need to think about how to answer questions when they are being asked.

Greg and Gina could use a preexisting coping mechanism, humor, as one solution to their dilemma. The familiarity of the coping mechanism eased their transition into dealing with questions and comments from a new perspective. When you observe strengths in your clients, you can use those strengths to help them, simply by encouraging them to adapt those strengths to a challenging situation. We have found that using our clients' preexisting strengths and coping mechanisms to develop strategies for problem solving often proves to be effective and efficient.

Dealing with Holidays and Family-Focused Celebrations

Many clients report experiencing an increase in the intensity of their infertility-related grief as the date of a holiday or family-focused celebration approaches. Clients describe grief responses as feelings of dread, increased isolation, hopelessness, and sadness. These grief reactions may turn holidays into events that mark yet another year that has passed the client by. Clients may also resent family and friends who are celebrating with or because of their children.

In clients' search for answers to understand or at least alleviate their grief symptoms, they often consider withdrawing from celebrations such as baby showers for coworkers or company picnics that include employees and their families. Clients may also weigh the implications of breaking with the established traditions of how the family celebrates significant holidays. These options will doubtless have consequences for the client; it is up to the client to determine the advantages and disadvantages of making these decisions.

We encourage clients to honor their need to decline invitations to events (such as a coworker's baby shower) that they view as extraneous to significant relationships. We also validate clients' prerogatives to establish boundaries and limits for their participation in established family traditions that cause them pain (such as Thanksgiving dinner with their siblings, nieces, and nephews). However, even as we encourage clients to honor their feelings, we also recommend that they think about how they may be able to influence their responses to these events. If clients can recognize that they are allowing their grief to dominate their view of celebrations, they may make decisions about participating in family events that are based on more than their grief responses. Simply put, an increase in self-awareness often leads to changes in perspective and behavior.

For instance, if you were working with a client who felt unable to attend her sister's baby shower because she felt it would only remind her of her own inability to get pregnant, you could talk with her about what her attendance at the shower or her decision not to go might mean to her sister. You could talk to her about the opportunity to share in her sister's joy and ask your client to consider what she would want her sister to do if the situation were reversed. You could also make a distinction between the significance of attending her sister's baby shower and attending a baby shower for a coworker. In the big picture, declining an invitation to a coworker's shower seems much less significant than choosing not to attend a sibling's baby shower. If after discussing these subjects your client decided not to go to her sister's shower, you might suggest that she discuss her decision with her sister and to be honest about her dilemma. Although clients need to honor their feelings about avoiding painful situations, they must also take into account the impact of their decisions on the relationships involved. They need to balance responding to their grief with responding to the needs of loved ones.

We should note that even though the increase in the intensity of the client's grief reaction may be perfectly justified, this reaction is not necessarily compatible with healthy functioning over the long term. Clients understandably may initially need to abstain from events that compound their grief. Eventually, however, clients who continue to withdraw from specific events may become more isolated and removed from potential sources of support. At some point, clients should be able to separate their grief from the celebrations of others and their own celebration of life's events. Otherwise, clients risk becoming critically stagnated in the grief process (for a more in-depth discussion of the warning signs and implications of stagnation in the grief process, see Chapter Five).

Coping with Others' Pregnancies

Women compose the majority of clients reporting difficulty coping with another's pregnancy. Although the male partner may also be struggling with his reactions to others' pregnancies, he usually reports that his difficulty relates more to his attempts to ease his partner's pain about this issue. This disparity makes sense when we consider the biological roles each gender plays in reproduction.

The man who is experiencing infertility loses the emotional experience that accompanies a pregnancy, whereas the woman loses both the emotional and physiological experience of pregnancy. Therefore, another person's pregnancy may become a symbol both of the couple's "failure" to have a child and of the woman's inability to *be* pregnant. This discussion is not intended to minimize a male partner's reaction to another couple's or person's pregnancy. As we work through our clients' feelings about other people who are expecting a biological child, we usually find that each partner is simply experiencing feelings related to the loss of the role (be it gender-specific or gender-neutral) that they would typically play during a pregnancy.

Clients frequently express their struggle with this issue by asking some form of the following question: "Why is it so difficult for me to see other people who are expecting a child, and how do I stop feeling so jealous of them?" For many clients experiencing infertility, the physical condition of pregnancy can become blatantly obvious. Clients regularly report that they feel as if everyone in the world is expecting a child, except for them. They may also perceive that a disproportionate number of women in their lives and in the public places they frequent are pregnant.

Clients often experience another couple's pregnancy from the perspective that pregnancy is symbolic of the client's own reproductive losses. Clients, both male and female, also tell us that they are frequently unable to feel any joy for other couples who are expecting a child. Furthermore, they tell us that most of the feelings that they do have about other expectant parents are "negative" feelings. These negative feelings may include jealousy, anger, impatience (especially as it relates to the pregnant woman's focus on her symptoms and complaints about discomfort and weight gain, the development of the fetus, and complaints that the couple's life will never be the same), animosity, and guilt (for having feelings that the client perceives as negative). The client who is experiencing these feelings is also likely to be experiencing a great deal of pain.

Most clients in this situation are fully aware that they need to address their feelings, but they are sometimes hesitant to risk exposing the intensity of their emotions for fear of being judged as a jealous, angry, and hostile person. Acknowledging these feelings requires already vulnerable clients to further lower their defenses and to risk eliciting the disapproval of others. However, not acknowledging these kinds of feelings, especially when they are directed toward people that our clients care about, can lead to distance in relationships and feelings of isolation from and resentment toward significant others in our clients' lives. When we work with clients who are feeling jealous or angry, we explain to them that although they need not acknowledge feelings of anger and jealousy with others at every turn, it is important for them to discuss their feelings, and to ask for support from the people they care about. We also point out that not everyone will be able to empathize with our clients' feelings, so clients must choose their support people carefully. We can offer support to our clients when they are trying to make a decision about discussing these emotions, because we recognize that they may be embroiled in a conflict between their desire to feel differently and their need for self-protection. Clients in this situation may feel as though they are between a rock and a hard place.

From a therapeutic perspective, you need to place these feelings into the context of grief and loss and validate them as understandable given the circumstances. However, you should also clearly explain to your clients that the answers to this dilemma will most likely be found within their own perceptions of their ability to respond in a different way. That is, clients profoundly strengthen their ability to directly influence their reactions when they have a genuine desire to change their behaviors, are willing to apply other successful coping mechanisms, and can acknowledge that they truly do have a choice about how they respond to any given situation. (Greg and Gina's decision to use humor as a coping mechanism, discussed earlier, illustrates this point.) It is our role to assist clients in expanding their perception of their abilities, and it is the client's role to use those abilities in her efforts to deal more effectively with the pregnancies of others.

Integrating One's Sexual History

As clients try to make sense of their experience with infertility, it is not unusual for them to question whether anything in their sexual history may have caused or contributed to the infertility. For instance, some sexually transmitted diseases (STDs) have been shown to cause or increase the risk of infertility. When clients who have fertility problems have also had one of these STDs, they may have feelings of guilt and responsibility for the infertility. Because there is nothing that our clients can do to change their sexual history or its influence on the fertility problems, they need to try to reconcile and integrate their feelings about their sexual history with their feelings about their present circumstances.

It can be particularly difficult when our clients' fertility problems are directly linked to an STD. However, the person who transmitted the STD, who may or may not be the client's life partner, is also partially responsible for the fertility problems. In these situations, little can be done to alleviate our clients' guilt beyond simply working through and accepting it. For our clients, it is a matter of acknowledging their responsibility and accepting that their guilt will not change their circumstances.

Clearly, we should not attempt to minimize the role the STD may have played in the fertility problems. Instead, we can focus on assisting our clients in accepting the reality of the situation and in finding a way for them to reconcile the issue for themselves and with their life partner. If the client's life partner cannot forgive the client for the client's role in the infertility, the couple may not be able to continue in the relationship. It is up to both partners in the relationship to decide whether or not they are willing and able to move beyond this issue. If both partners are willing to work on the guilt or resentment that may arise from an STD being the cause of fertility problems, we would suggest that additional work be done on these issues before proceeding with further infertility counseling. In these situations we might adapt the Special Concerns session (see Chapter Ten) to address these issues with our clients. We might also ask clients to postpone further treatment or investigation into parenting alternatives until they are able to reconcile these issues in their relationship and integrate them into the entire infertility experience. You should know the circumstances under which your client contracted the STD: Was the STD contracted prior to the marriage? During the marriage? Did the client know about the STD prior to the infertility diagnosis, and was the client honest with her partner about it? Any marital work should be done in the context of those circumstances. The circumstances are relevant because they will influence the issues that the couple will need to discuss.

Another issue that arises in conjunction with infertility and our clients' sexual histories has to do with the relationship between a previous abortion and fertility problems. When your clients are confronted with infertility and the potential loss of the biological child, a previous abortion may take on new meaning for them. In the following passage, Rebecca explores her feelings about a previous abortion, describing them from a pre- and post-infertility perspective:

Before we were diagnosed with infertility, I had never really had any regrets about my decision to terminate my pregnancy. I felt like I had made the only decision that I could make, given my circumstances at the time. After we were diagnosed with infertility, I started to wonder if that was the only pregnancy I would ever experience.

It's so strange how a pregnancy can mean so many different things to the same person at different points in her life. With the pregnancy that I terminated, being pregnant was really scary and I felt totally overwhelmed. Now here I am, desperately trying to get pregnant. Now a pregnancy seems like it would be the answer to all of my problems. I know it really wouldn't be, but infertility treatment is so goal-focused that reaching the goal of pregnancy seems like the ultimate success.

Sometimes I wonder if I blew my only chance to have biological kids. Then, I remember what kind of life we would have had if I had carried that pregnancy to term. There is just no going back. I suppose I would make the same decisions all over again, but the infertility adds another layer of perspective to the choices I have made. I guess one of those layers is grief about the lost opportunity to be a parent. And another one is grief for the lost child, the one that might have been and the ones I have lost through infertility.

From Rebecca's description of her circumstances, we can see that she was struggling with the differences between the meaning that pregnancy once had and the meaning that pregnancy now had for her. We worked with Rebecca on the differences between the meaning the abortion once had for her and the meaning the abortion had taken on in her life. Rebecca's predicament was further complicated because she had been raped, and the pregnancy that she terminated was a result of this sexual assault. All these issues—the infertility, the abortion, and the sexual assault—had to be dealt with for her to begin to recover from her losses and the ensuing grief. Ultimately, she was able to accept her past decisions, grieve for all her losses, and integrate both her pre- and post-infertility perspectives into her present identity. It was this integration that allowed her to move forward in her quest to parent. (For more information about our work with Rebecca, see the Special Concerns session in Chapter Ten.)

Because sexuality and infertility are inextricably intertwined, therapists who are working with clients who have fertility problems will also be working with issues about their clients' sexual history and its newfound relationship to the infertility. (For more information on sexuality and infertility, please see Chapter Six.) Some clients will struggle anew with issues they may have viewed as resolved or in-significant. Thus, after a diagnosis of infertility, clients' sexual histories may take on new meaning for them and their life partner. Clients' integrating the new meaning of these experiences into their identity allows them to move toward self-actualization.

Accepting the Parenting Practices of Others

When clients are struggling to fulfill their desire to become parents, they are often acutely aware of the parenting styles and child-rearing practices of other parents. Clients frequently discuss their perspectives on the parenting practices of friends and family members. They often choose to discuss the most extreme examples of harmful parenting. In relaying these examples to us, clients appear mystified as to how these parents can treat their children so badly.

These clients seem to have the most difficulty with media reports of child abuse and neglect. They often ask us, "Why is it, when we want a child so badly and can't have one, that these people who are unfit to be parents can have children?" Clients tell us that they cannot understand why God would give children to "those" people but not to them, especially when it is obvious to the clients who the better parents would be. They also express their wonder at why nature has played such a dirty trick on them. However they express this concept, the one word clients use over and over again to describe their feelings on this issue is *unfair.*

Clients' sense of fair play is clearly shaping the meaning they have given to this aspect of their experience: it is not fair to us that we want a child, are prepared to parent, and cannot have a child, when so many people that have them are not prepared to parent and are not doing a very good job. We contend that when clients attempt to understand infertility through their definition of what is *fair,* they are trying to fit the proverbial square peg into a round hole. Considering that reproduction is dependent on a multitude of physiological factors and that sexual behavior and contraception are subject to the free agency of each individual, equity or fairness has nothing to do with who becomes a biological parent and who does not.

We share this perspective with our clients in a gentle and caring way, but we also emphasize the inevitably random nature of infertility, because we know that when our clients are focused on the unfairness of their situation, they are expressing their grief through anger.

It may very well be unfair that others are able to parent, adequately or inadequately, but focusing on fairness will not change our clients' circumstances. We try to help our clients express their grief in ways that will lead them to acceptance of the infertility. Dealing with their grief on a more personal level will not change the infertility diagnosis either, but it may help our clients respond to their circumstances in a more effective way.

When clients who are outraged by the prevalence of child abuse and neglect want to act on their concerns for children, we suggest that they get involved in an organization that advocates on behalf of children. For some clients, volunteering, foster-parenting abused children, or participating in an advocacy organization on behalf of children may help them find new meaning in their infertility experience and help children at the same time. This shift in perspective is another example of clients' empowering themselves by taking responsibility for the effect that life's circumstances will have on them. Clients can either focus on the injustice of infertility or act to alleviate the injustice around them. For many, the decision to act enables them to derive meaning from their suffering.

CRISIS

When clients are confronted with one or several of the dilemmas raised in the previous discussion, these dilemmas can compound the initial grief reaction to the diagnosis of infertility. The resulting combination of experiences can catapult individuals into a full-blown life crisis and cause them to feel paralyzed by their circumstances.

For many clients infertility is an unexpected loss; they may experience receiving the diagnosis and undergoing infertility treatment as a personal crisis, one that puts them at a difficult crossroad. These clients subsequently often behave in ways that are not characteristic of their usual ways of functioning. They bear the challenge of conquering the crisis that can result from diagnosis and treatment, and then the challenge of integrating into their identity the loss of what fertility represents, without their usual repertoire of coping skills. Clients who struggle with a crisis brought on by an infertility diagnosis can take one of several paths: they may take a road that leads them straight through to the integration of infertility into their identities, by way of acceptance. We have also seen clients detoured and plummeted onto traumatic paths before they reach integration.

Acceptance

As we have said, some clients are able to accept the condition of infertility and to integrate the experience into their identities with little turmoil. They are then able to explore other parenting alternatives rationally and easily. These clients do not feel as though their world has been turned upside down, nor are they in a state of denial about their infertility diagnosis. We usually see these clients in treatment for consultations about specific parenting alternatives and appropriate courses of action.

Clients who are not devastated by their circumstances are usually capable of accepting the condition of infertility for a variety of reasons, and they can explain their response to the diagnosis in understandable terms. Some people know, before they attempt to bear children, that their medical conditions may render a pregnancy very risky. Others, through positive exposure to child-free couples, blended families, and adopted children, are readily able to consider alternatives to biological parenting. And still others, some of whom are medical professionals themselves, refuse to be subjected to the known side effects of treatment. Some people, for practical reasons, choose not to use their financial resources on the gamble of infertility treatment, and instead proceed with adoption as a better guarantee of parenting. And we have had highly religious clients who view their infertility as a blessing in disguise, as it freed them to respond to the children already waiting for homes.

Because the infertility diagnosis comes after unsuccessful attempts to have biological children on their own, these clients usually pursue alternatives to biological parenting pragmatically and easily. What all these reactions have in common is that the primary objective in each scenario is *parenting,* not *biological* parenting.

Although acceptance of an infertility condition with little turmoil may not be common, it is a healthy response. We highlight this response in order to represent both ends of the spectrum of responses. At the other end of the spectrum are clients who receive an infertility diagnosis and subsequent treatment and respond by feeling completely devastated and powerless. Because we intended this book to help clients who are experiencing difficulty with integrating the infertility experience into their identity, we need to examine the trauma our clients can experience on their journey toward that integration.

Trauma

Trauma can be caused by a painful emotional experience or by a bodily injury, wound, or shock; clients dealing with infertility can experience both kinds of trauma. First, the loss of the opportunity to parent biological children can be such a shock to clients that they are unable to incorporate the news of their predicament in a manner consistent with their typical way of coping. (This denial, which is part of grief, is discussed in Chapter Five.) Second, the treatment for infertility is often invasive and painful, particularly if it occurs over a long period of time. Clients experiencing infertility as a trauma must adapt to their predicament, or they are at risk for experiencing Posttraumatic Stress Disorder (PTSD).

PTSD is usually recognized and diagnosed through a distinct group of coping mechanisms. For the purposes of this discussion, we will explain the *DSM-IV* criteria for PTSD as they might relate to a client's experience of infertility.

1. The client has been exposed to a traumatic event and has experienced a threat to his physical integrity, and the client's response involves intense fear, helplessness, or horror. Infertility can be perceived as a threat to a client's physical integrity. Integrity is the quality or state of being complete, unbroken, and whole. Because the human body was designed to procreate, and being fertile is the "unbroken" condition of the body, one could reason that a body that is not fertile is in a "broken condition" or without integrity. Furthermore, the client may feel helpless to change his condition and fearful of the long-term implications of the infertility. These fears might include fear of not fitting into the broader culture, of being left out of family-centered events, of marital dissolution or distress, and of diminishing self-worth. As the client initially responds to the infertility diagnosis, infertility is often perceived as a life-changing force that leads clients to begin asking, "Why is this happening to me?"

2. The traumatic event is continuously relived as intense psychological distress when the client is exposed to cues that symbolize an aspect of the trauma. As the diagnosis of infertility sinks in and a client pursues treatment, she may find herself in a cycle of enthusiastic expectation, wait-and-see, and then disappointment when treatment is unsuccessful. Each time the client rides the cycle of infertility treatment, she may reexperience the physical, emotional, and psychological

anxiety she encountered during the previous cycle. In addition, cues such as seeing a pregnant woman or receiving an invitation to a baby shower might symbolize the persistent failure to procreate. These experiences and perceptions may cause clients to ask questions to which no one can truthfully reply, such as "How much longer will we have to undergo treatment before we get pregnant?" and "What is God's plan for me?"

3. The client persistently avoids stimuli associated with the trauma, as indicated by feelings of detachment or estrangement from others; avoidance of activities, places, or people that arouse recollections of the trauma; and a sense of a foreshortened future. As discussed elsewhere, many clients withdraw from social settings in order to avoid participating in conversations that may trigger the experience of infertility. Clients also may report feeling a sense of doom about their future and ask, "What if the treatment doesn't work?" and "What will my life mean without children?"

4. The client has persistent symptoms of increased arousal, as indicated by irritability and difficulty concentrating. Some clients report that they become so preoccupied with their treatment, monthly cycles, and the desire to become biological parents that they no longer find meaning in the things that were once worthwhile. Sometimes, a well-intentioned "How are you?" from a friend or family member causes the client to become irritated or angry because the answer to the question is exasperating and depressing. Clients may begin to ask, "How can people be so insensitive?" and "Why am I so edgy these days?"

5. The disturbance lasts more than one month. Many of our clients report that the disturbance begins with the infertility diagnosis and intensifies with prolonged medical treatment. They add that the intensity of the psychological symptoms remain even after they have discontinued medical treatment. Many clients tell us they have difficulty finding meaning in the persistent failure of medical interventions to produce a viable pregnancy, and they wonder, "How much more of this can I take?"

6. The disturbance causes clinically significant distress or impairment in social, occupational, or other important areas of functioning. Many clients report that their infertility diagnosis has left them incapable of functioning normally. Some clients feel as if the world is going on without them, and no one seems to notice that they have been left behind. Many clients become so distressed by their plight that they question the meaning of all the choices they have made up

to this point in their lives. They may wonder if they made the right choice of spouse, career, past sexual behavior, and timing for family planning. (Reprinted with permission from the *Diagnostic and Statistical Manual of Mental Disorders, Fourth Edition.* Copyright © 1994, American Psychiatric Association)

———

Clients who experience infertility as a trauma and exhibit the associated symptoms of PTSD may feel that their life is meaningless, that everything is hopeless; these clients' functioning is severely impaired. In these circumstances, you should incorporate a traditional trauma model into your therapeutic approach. This includes supporting your clients while they relive the traumatic events, let go of the self-blame, grieve, rediscover their inner self, and integrate the traumatic experience into the whole of their life experience. (You might also consider using Judith Lewis Herman's *Trauma and Recovery* as a guide.)

PART THREE

Strategies for Treatment

〰 *Misfortunes do not flourish particularly in our path.*
They grow everywhere.
   —*Big Elk, Omaha chief,* Cherokee Feast of Days

P art Three includes Chapters Five through Nine. Chapter Five, "Coping with Reproductive Loss," discusses the impact of reproductive losses, the stages of grief for clients experiencing infertility, and treatment strategies for dealing with specific reproductive losses. Chapter Six, "Dealing with Sexuality and Infertility," examines the influence that infertility has on clients' sexuality. Chapter Seven, "Considering Alternatives to Biological Parenting," looks at the issues that confront clients who are considering parenting through a donor alternative or adoption, or who are considering child-free living. Chapter Eight, "Coping with Recurring Grief and Doubt," identifies specific events that may trigger a resurgence of grief at any point during the client's life cycle. Chapter Nine, "Regaining a Healthy Identity," summarizes our philosophy and connects our treatment strategies to the concept of integrating infertility into the client's identity. All of these chapters include cases, treatment strategies for specific issues, and strategies for using the exercises provided in Chapter Eleven.

CHAPTER FIVE

Coping with Reproductive Loss

Only through mourning everything that she has lost can the patient discover her indestructible inner life.

—*Judith Lewis Herman,* Trauma and Recovery

In Chapter Three we discussed the relationships among infertility and functioning, identity, and gender, and how all are linked by the common theme of loss. In this chapter, we explore *reproductive losses*: those experienced by clients diagnosed with infertility and those that ultimately may not fit into the "textbook" definition of infertility (the inability to conceive within one year by a couple who is having consistent intercourse). For our purposes, the expression *clients who are experiencing infertility* includes clients who are experiencing fertility problems. For instance, some of our clients initially experience difficulty carrying a pregnancy to term, have one or more miscarriages, and then are able to experience a normal pregnancy. Others have difficulty conceiving, pursue medical treatment, and then are able to achieve a pregnancy without further intervention. Still others have difficulty conceiving, pursue medical treatment, and are still unable to have biological children.

Whether your clients have had difficulty conceiving or difficulty carrying a pregnancy to term, all will have experienced reproductive losses. Reproductive losses are losses associated with conception and pregnancy and include miscarriages, stillbirths, and the loss of the *potential biological child* through the inability to achieve a pregnancy. Clearly, not all people who experience a reproductive loss will ultimately be unable to have biological children. However, even if they do not fit the textbook definition of infertility, clients who have experienced a reproductive loss can benefit from grief therapy. Therefore, the information in this chapter is intended to help you in your work with all clients who have experienced reproductive losses. We begin by identifying the cultural context in which our clients experience reproductive losses, because the context influences our clients' perceptions about what is *lost*. We then explore the impact of reproductive losses, discuss the process of grieving reproductive losses, and conclude with a discussion on differentiating between and working with specific reproductive losses.

EXPLORING CULTURAL ATTITUDES

Cultural attitudes about pregnancy and childbirth guide the development of our individual values, attitudes, and ideas about reproduction. Cultural attitudes also set the standards for behavior and influence the ways in which people respond to pregnancy, childbirth, and the loss of fertility. Culturally speaking, reproduction has been given intrinsic meaning in virtually every aspect of human experience, and therefore a vast array of attitudes about reproduction have evolved.

Regardless of how we label a particular cultural attitude about reproduction, we need to remember that societal expectations can be based on morality, customs influenced by biological theories, and so on. First and foremost among all cultural attitudes is the societal expectation that all humans will participate in reproduction. Reproduction for the continuation of our species is not only an implied responsibility of each person but also assumed to be an entitlement. People who are exempt from this expectation include some members of the clergy and individuals with genetic disorders or life-threatening medical conditions. There also are exceptions based on *malice or misunderstanding* (or both), for people who can be perceived as unsuitable for parenting or as inferior (people with disabilities, welfare mothers, and lesbians and gay men, for example).

Following are lists of some of the cultural attitudes (standards for behavior, values, and ideas) that surround reproduction. Cultural attitudes may be held as "truths" (and we have written them here as pronouncements of those truths), but it is important to remember that they are in fact judgments, beliefs, and assumptions.

Societal Expectations
- All humans will participate in reproduction.
- Reproduction is a function of marriage.
- Pregnant women must act in the best interest of the fetus.
- Once one enters this realm of responsibility, one will be required to make personal sacrifices for the benefit of one's children.

Moral Principles
- Pregnancy and childbirth are proof of irresponsibility when parents are "too young" or financially and emotionally unprepared for parenthood.
- Pregnancy and children are a manifestation of God's grace.
- The birth of a child is a miracle, and the parents' role in the process is equal to participation in a genesis.

Customs
- Under all of the "right" circumstances, pregnancy and childbirth are cause for celebration.
- Educating new parents through classes on childbirth, books on parenting, and instructions on proper prenatal care is essential.
- Labor and delivery are rites of passage into parenthood.
- The experience of labor and delivery is essential to the bonding process between parents and their child.
- It is perfectly acceptable for strangers or near-strangers to put their hands on a pregnant woman's stomach.

Theories of Biology as Destiny
- Pregnancy is the biological destiny of women.
- To impregnate is the biological destiny of men.
- Children represent a biological extension of self and the continuation of the genetic family line.
- Children are the parents' contribution to the future of the human race.
- Childbirth is a demonstration of membership in the human community.
- Reproduction ensures the parents' immortality.

We should note that the beliefs derived from the idea of biology as destiny stem from reproduction's being essential to the survival of the human species. Nature defines the biological roles of men and women in the reproductive process, and the validity of those roles is not at issue here. What is at issue is the idea that men and women must want or be able to procreate in order to be of value to our species. It is this idea that interferes with the ability of clients who are experiencing infertility to define their value as a human being.

Although not all of the specific customs, attitudes, morals, and theories that we have listed here relate directly to infertility, they all demonstrate the influence that our values and attitudes about pregnancy and childbirth have on our behaviors and opinions. For instance, the custom of asking after a pregnant woman's health and patting her stomach as a way of acknowledging the pregnancy does not have anything to do with infertility. It does, however, have to do with the assumptions we automatically make about pregnancy. We assume, first of all, that the woman is comfortable with this very personal gesture, and second, that our concern for the baby's well-being entitles us to touch someone in a manner that under any other circumstances would be considered forward and inappropriate. Like many of the assumptions we make about pregnancy and childbirth, the assumption that it is acceptable to touch a pregnant woman's stomach has nothing to do with the individual woman's boundaries but has to do with *our* assumptions about what is true.

RECOGNIZING THE IMPACT OF REPRODUCTIVE LOSSES

As we have discussed, our clients' experience of infertility will be directly influenced by the cultural significance of pregnancy and childbirth. The significance of reproduction to humans is evidenced by the sheer number of attitudes but also by our fascination with reproduction. For instance, the mating rituals of virtually every accessible species on this planet are subject to scientific investigation. As humans, we are fascinated by the similarities and differences between our reproductive habits and those of other species. We are also fascinated by the similarities and differences between the reproductive habits of various human subcultures. We study, compare, write, film, sculpt, paint, pretend, rejoice, imagine, worship, ritualize, celebrate, and marry, all in the name of reproduction. Perhaps it is the "miracle" of reproduction or our desire to participate in creation that leads to part of our fascination. Whatever the cause, reproduction—pregnancy and childbirth—is central to our identity as human beings.

We have identified three primary ways that our clients are affected after they have experienced fertility problems. Our clients tell us that infertility and the accompanying reproductive losses they experience engender feelings of isolation, of powerlessness, and of deprivation. The next sections of our discussion explore these three areas of impact on our clients.

Isolation

Because reproduction is central to our human identity, clients who are confronting infertility may feel *outside* one of the most human of experiences. Clients may also find that the cultural expressions of the significance of pregnancy and childbirth serve as painful reminders of their exclusion from these most basic human experiences. For instance, clients who are experiencing infertility may still feel obliged to attend a baby shower for another couple or a naming ceremony for a newborn. Our clients tell us that these culturally sanctioned celebrations of pregnancy and childbirth sometimes foster their sense of isolation from the culture at large.

The following case illustrates how one couple, Nancy and Jason, revealed their sense of isolation as they dealt with cultural celebrations of reproduction and their infertility diagnosis.

NANCY: One of my college friends was in town this week, and on Saturday her mother had a baby shower for her. I was really excited about seeing her and some of my other old friends, and I guess I just didn't think about what it might be like for me to see her pregnant. I mean, I wondered what she would look like pregnant, but it didn't occur to me to think about whether or not I would have a negative reaction.

When I walked in the door, I immediately noticed that two of the other guests were pregnant. I couldn't believe it, but I felt like I was going to start crying. It was so weird. Anyway, I walked in and as soon as I saw my friend, her name is Julia, we just started hugging each other and both of us were crying. I was really aware of the fact that part of why I was crying had to do with being sad. So when we finally calmed down a little, she started introducing me to the other women at the shower. One of the women she introduced to me was pregnant, and for the first time I noticed that she was drinking a glass of wine. I just couldn't stop staring at her. I think my mouth was probably hanging open and the look on my face . . . well, I don't know, but I think it might have been obvious that I was shocked. She, the pregnant wine-drinker, just acted like nothing was happening. So I guess I must have closed my mouth and then I took my gift over to the table.

So here I am, sitting in what seems to be a room full of pregnant women, and I am just sitting there with nothing to say. Well, plenty to say, but I couldn't say any of it. Everyone else in the room is sharing labor and delivery stories and I just felt totally out of place. Then one of the other women asked me whether or not I had any kids, and even though I said no in a very polite way, I was feeling really angry at her for asking me such an insensitive question. Julia knows about the miscarriage, so she just looked at me in a supportive kind of way. It was nice of her, but I just couldn't help thinking that she could be supportive from now until tomorrow and it wouldn't change the fact that she has no idea what I have gone through.

THERAPIST: Nancy, it seems to me that some of your emotions were fostered by your beliefs about what it means to be pregnant. For instance, you said that you felt as though you did not fit in with the other guests and had nothing to contribute to their conversation. Part of your reaction may have been based on not wanting to cry or discuss the miscarriage at the baby shower, but your reaction may also have been based on a belief that says that since you have not been able to carry a pregnancy to term you have nothing of value to say to others who have or who are about to carry a pregnancy to term. What do you think?

NANCY: I do feel that way. Even though it may sound crazy I felt like I couldn't say anything to the wine-drinking woman about the dangers of alcohol. I couldn't say anything because I feel like, who am I to tell her how to have a healthy baby? I can't have one, so I'm obviously not the expert. And during the labor and delivery discussion, what was I supposed to say? Having a miscarriage is also a very difficult experience? Can you imagine?

THERAPIST: You know, discussing the miscarriage may not have been appropriate, but not having carried a pregnancy to term does not necessarily mean that you don't know anything about pregnancy. It seems that you have equated the inability to have a child with an inability to offer anything of value on the subject of pregnancy. Although it may not have been your role to confront the "wine drinker," it doesn't mean that alcohol has not been shown to have detrimental effects on a developing fetus. You have strong beliefs about prenatal health, and it seems to me that you are entitled to those beliefs regardless of the infertility. However, you are feeling like the inability to have a child and the loss of your role as a mother makes you or your opinions less valuable. Can you see how those feelings may be based on the cultural belief that women must *be able* to be mothers in order to have any *real* value in this society?

NANCY: I think so. So you're saying that I have started to put less value on myself as a woman or a person because I can't have a child?

THERAPIST: That is how it sounds to me. What do you think?

NANCY: I think that is true, because I am always feeling unsure of what I have to offer. I hesitate before I offer my opinions, especially when it comes to children and pregnancy, and I rarely offer those opinions to people who know about the infertility or the miscarriage. I guess I do that because I think they will ignore my advice because they think I can't possibly know what I am talking about. You know, because of the miscarriage.

UNDERSTANDING THE SOURCE OF EMOTIONS.   Although helping Nancy to see the connections between her reactions, her values, and societal attitudes about fertility did not eliminate her emotions, it did help her understand where some of her emotions were coming from. Once she understood the source of some of the emotions, we were able to identify several examples of how cultural attitudes were influencing her reactions and to reevaluate the relevance of those attitudes to her life. We did this simply by talking about what she really believed about herself and what she thought she *should* believe about herself. For instance, when we discussed Nancy's value as a woman we talked about all the things about her that are valuable, in spite of the infertility diagnosis. Ultimately, Nancy began to separate her value as a woman and a person from the idea that she had to procreate in order to be valuable.

DEALING WITH FEELINGS OF ISOLATION.   Nancy described feelings during this session that are similar to those described by other clients we counsel about infertility issues. There are no easy answers to the questions Nancy is asking herself. In our work with Nancy and Jason, we subsequently focused on trying to find some of those answers. For instance, this couple wanted to prepare themselves for future situations like the baby shower. We worked on anticipating events that would pose a problem and making decisions about whether to attend or to decline the invitations. We also discussed the benefits of having prepared answers to questions about children, pregnancy, and parenting. Prepared answers eliminate the need to think about how to answer questions when they are being asked.

Jason and Nancy's ideas about their obligation to attend a baby shower or to fully answer questions about their status as parents were based on their beliefs that they had to participate in child-focused celebrations and that they owed others an explanation for their nonparticipation in reproduction. As we took a closer look at Nancy and Jason's beliefs about childbirth and pregnancy and identified the attitudes that were influencing their behavior, they discovered that some of their beliefs were based on nothing more than habit and cultural influence. This discovery had a tremendous impact on their ability to cope with the infertility and their ultimate decision to explore alternatives to biological parenting.

Not all clients experiencing infertility have the same reactions to cultural attitudes, because clients have different personal beliefs and values. In the therapeutic setting, we must first ascertain what the client's culture, values, customs, and beliefs about reproduction are. We are then better able to understand how losing something they value, such as the ability to be biological parents, might affect them.

Accepting the Limitations of Infertility

Infertility limits an individual's reproductive capability and usually requires medical intervention to increase the possibility of conception. Therefore, clients experiencing infertility must make reproductive decisions based on the limits that infertility puts on their reproductive functions and in accordance with the medical plan for treatment. Clients thus lose some of their capacity to act independently in making those reproductive decisions. Even if clients choose not to pursue medical intervention, they are still limited by the physiological implications of infertility. In other words, infertility imposes an additional set of rules on reproduction: clients are still free to choose their course of action, but infertility limits the courses of action they have to choose from.

Furthermore, because of their infertility, clients must rely on the skill of medical professionals, the odds of success with reproductive technologies, and their bodies' ability to respond to interventions. Clearly, the influence that clients had or believed they had over reproduction is severely limited. It is worth repeating, however, that how clients *respond* to their diagnosis is still very much within their influence.

Jake reflected on the sense of powerlessness he and Kristi felt in the face of all these limitations:

> Kristi and I had been married for three years when we decided we were ready to have kids. Before that we had been really careful about preventing a pregnancy, because we just didn't feel we were ready. After we decided to start a family we tried for about two years before we went to a specialist. After all the tests had been taken and analyzed our doctor told us that Kristi wasn't ovulating and that I had a low sperm count.
>
> I can't tell you how disappointed we were. We had been under the illusion that we would go off of the birth control and be able to get pregnant. We just couldn't believe that we would have to go through all these complicated treatments, take medication, and possibly undergo surgical procedures in order to have a child. And even then there wouldn't be any guarantees. It was so disorienting. I mean we just felt like the rug had been pulled out from under us. One minute we were preventing a pregnancy, and the next minute we were being told that technology would determine whether or not we would be able to have biological kids. At this point, we feel like we don't have any control over whether or not we become parents.

Jake was struggling with his desire to have a biological child and his realization that his and Kristi's medical problems might be barriers to fulfilling that desire. As Jake's level of influence over fulfilling his and Kristi's desire to have a child diminished and the influence of external factors over their fate as potential parents increased, Jake's feelings of powerlessness also increased.

To help Jake and Kristi deal with their sense of powerlessness, we talked with them about their ability to make certain choices. We began by making a distinction between the ability to have biological children and the ability to fulfill their desire to become parents. We also talked with them about their ability to decide whether or not they would continue to pursue biological parenting. We acknowledged that the infertility diagnosis was certainly going to limit their ability to get pregnant, but we also tried to help them see that they were not left without any choices or influence over becoming parents.

We talked to them about the reproductive technologies that were available to them, the option of child-free living, and adoption. In discussing these options, Jake and Kristi began to make choices about the options that might be right for them. By acknowledging their sense of powerlessness and discussing the choices that were still available to them, we helped Jake and Kristi to accept both the limitations that biology had imposed and the shift in the degree of influence they had over reproduction.

Deprivation

Infertility oftentimes deprives our clients of the experiences of pregnancy, childbirth, and biological parenting. As our clients discuss the loss of these experiences, their descriptions of their feelings are marked by a profound sense of abandonment. They feel abandoned by their bodies, by their ability to achieve their goals, by God, and by friends and family who seem unable to understand the depth of our clients' loss. Our clients also tell us that they feel they are being deprived of the opportunity to give their love to a child, pass on their genetic heritage, and to experience the joys and sorrows of parenthood.

When we work with clients around their feelings of deprivation, we begin by validating their feelings. Indeed, infertility may very well deprive our clients of the experience of biological parenting. As the opening epigraph of this chapter confirms, it is only by mourning all our losses that we are able to discover "our indestructible inner lives."

Therefore, we must acknowledge our clients' sense of deprivation in order to facilitate the healing process. We do this by encouraging our clients to name their losses and to explore the meaning that their losses will have for them. For example, if a client tells us that he feels deprived of the experience of passing on his genetic heritage, we ask him to explore what it means to him to miss that experience. Although we may eventually make suggestions about how our clients can pass on a part of themselves through adoptive parenting or making contributions that will enrich the lives of children who are not their direct descendants (through charitable organizations or foster parenting), we do not expect that acting on these suggestions will or should retract our clients' previous losses. Instead, we offer these suggestions as a way of helping our clients find meaning in their lives that may restore their sense of wholeness and add to their identity as a human being, despite the losses they have experienced.

GRIEVING AND REPRODUCTIVE LOSSES

Throughout this book we discuss grief and its relationship to infertility. All clients who are experiencing infertility will experience a grief reaction: with infertility comes loss, and with loss comes grief. However, many clients do not recognize their grief as such because they do not feel they are allowed to grieve for a child they never had or the biological parents they will not be. So first we work with our clients to help them understand the importance of grieving.

Acknowledging the Importance of Grieving

Each client's situation is different, and taking a thorough client history can help you assess the client's needs. The history should include information about the client's infertility treatment and outcomes, details on any pregnancies, miscarriages, stillbirths, or reproductive surgeries, and the client's original and subsequent reactions to the loss of potential biological children. You can use many of the exercises found in Chapter Eleven to assist you in gathering this information. You can use the couples inventory, for example, to assess (1) the intensity of the impact of the infertility on each partner in the relationship, (2) the similarities and differences between each partner's perception of the impact of the infertility, and (3) any significant discrepancies between how one partner *says* he feels and how the other partner *thinks* he feels.

You can also use the personal loss inventory, which asks clients to name their losses and discuss the impact of those losses. The purpose of this exercise is to provide both you and the client with insight into the client's history of loss, how past losses may be affecting the client's perspective on her reproductive losses, how the client copes with loss over time, and how the client has integrated previous losses into her present identity. You can ask clients to focus on their reproductive losses when they are filling out this form or to address loss in general.

When you review this form you should be looking for connections between past and present losses and any impact that previous losses may be having on your client's experience with infertility. When you discuss this form with your clients you can also ask them to describe any connections that they are aware of between previous and present losses.

When reviewing the personal loss inventory, you will also want to ask about any self-destructive patterns of coping, such as a reliance on alcohol or drugs, withdrawal from significant relationships, suicide attempts, or drastic changes in eating or sleep patterns. You can ask clients to fill out the form using a general perspective or to complete the exercise with infertility as the focus. These questionnaires can be helpful at any point during clients' experience with infertility, even if they are ten years beyond their original diagnosis of infertility.

Guiding Clients Through the Grief Process

The intensity of the grief response will vary from client to client, and clients will cope with grief in many different ways. However, we have found the following model of the stages of grief (first developed by Elizabeth Kübler-Ross) to be generally applicable to most of our clients. We have adapted her five stages of grief to reflect our clients' experiences. We use this model both to guide our assessment and to develop treatment plans.

STAGE ONE: DENIAL AND SHOCK.   Clients are often in this stage before they seek medical treatment—denial often manifests as postponed investigation of difficulties with conception—and again after an infertility problem or diagnosis is confirmed. During this stage your clients may be in shock about the infertility diagnosis and may be unable to consider the possibility that they may be unable to have biological children. Clients in this stage of grief often say things like "This cannot be happening to me" and "I'm sure there must be some kind of mistake. I just can't believe that we aren't going to be able to have children."

Clients in this stage of grief will repeatedly postpone going to a specialist and refuse to take diagnostic tests. This reaction is often based on the hope that something will change; postponing a diagnosis allows clients to delay facing the reality of their loss. Your clients may also report that they feel numb, or they will say things like "I don't know how I feel," or "I don't feel anything." Feelings of disbelief or numbness are an expected part of the process of grieving.

It is hard to say what an appropriate amount of time is for this stage to last, as all clients deal with loss differently. However, clients may engage in certain behaviors that serve as warning signs that they are "stuck" in this stage of grief: throwing themselves into their work and refusing to look at their pain, immediately pursuing an adoption because they believe that adopting a child will resolve their feelings of loss, using alcohol or drugs to sustain their lack of feeling or numbness, or increasingly relying on alcohol, sex, food, or prescription drugs to cope with their feelings of grief.

Clients may also begin Stage Three of the grief process—bargaining and negotiating—while still in Stage One. For instance, they may be in denial and at the same time begin bargaining in order to delay accepting that there may be a physical barrier to conception, one that may not be resolvable. Clients who are in these two stages simultaneously may get three or four medical opinions about the causes of their difficulties with conception or may continually postpone surgical procedures or starting medication. As we mentioned earlier, some couples may immediately look into adoption rather than acknowledge that they need to grieve before they can move on to alternatives for parenting.

Some of your clients may automatically assume that their fertility problems are part of God's plan (which in and of itself is not a reason for concern). However, this perspective can be a problem if clients relinquish all control to a greater being and deny that the losses are painful, or if clients tell you they feel fine about turning over their fate without acknowledging that acceptance of infertility is a process and that grief is part of that process.

STAGE TWO: ANGER AND ANGUISH. Clients in this stage are often feeling deep anguish over the possibility that they may never experience biological parenting. Clients often feel angry because they think it is unfair that they cannot have children and that life continues to go forward in spite of their pain. They may be angry at their bodies for failing them. They may feel jealousy over other people's pregnancies, question the parenting practices of others, experience discomfort in social situations, feel that their gender identity is being compromised by their diagnosis, or experience a combination of these feelings.

Clients in this stage of the grief process can be defensive and angry at the world for the injustice of the infertility. They may isolate themselves from others because they feel that nobody understands their pain and that other people cannot deal with their anger. During this stage, sex can become a reminder of their reproductive losses or the inability to conceive a child. Clients may also feel and express resentment toward their partner because they believe that their partner does not understand their feelings and problems or does not seem to feel as bad as they do.

Many of the difficulties that develop between couples who are experiencing infertility begin during this stage of the grief process. Communication issues that were manageable in the past become unmanageable or seemingly unresolvable. Clients in this stage often misdirect their anger or feelings of helplessness at their partner, causing their relationship to suffer.

Many of our clients in this stage also ask such questions as "Why is God punishing me?" "What is the meaning of my life without children?" and "Why is life so unfair?" Clients may also question their value as a person; feel that they have no value as a man, or woman, or potential parent; and say things like "I feel empty" (or broken, useless, or damaged).

STAGE THREE: BARGAINING AND NEGOTIATING.   During this stage our clients often try to negotiate with whatever force they think has control over human destiny. For example, people who believe in God might promise to live better lives if they can have biological children. They do this in hopes of making sense out of their predicament or finding answers that will change things.

During this stage, clients may intensify medical interventions and treatment for the infertility. In some of these cases, clients are trying to bargain with technology in order to change the outcome of their diagnosis. Clients in this stage may also pursue as many options as possible: adoption, in vitro fertilization, surrogacy, and so on.

The grief process frequently stagnates when clients are in this stage. By continuing to pursue treatment or bargain with "the forces that be," clients may feel that they are keeping the possibility of biological parenting alive. Clients may manifest stagnation in this stage of grief through an obsessive pursuit of medical treatment or an intense need to find a way to alter the results of their medical condition. Clients may say things like "If only I had done X, things might have been different" or "What if we stop trying, and the next attempt was the one that was going to work?" or "We should have made different choices along the way, and maybe we should reconsider the path we have chosen." This questioning of the possibilities and attempting to reconstruct the outcomes of medical treatment are examples of bargaining in hindsight through wishful thinking.

In this stage, clients' feelings that a pregnancy is the answer to problems in the marriage may strongly intensify. Clients may begin to
think that if only they could get pregnant, all the issues in their marriage would magically disappear. They may believe that getting pregnant would mean that their pain would stop, that they would no
longer feel inadequate as a life partner, that they would resolve their
resentment of their partner's "lack of understanding," or that the grief
that is a part of their sexual relationship would go away. These clients
are striking bargains between their bodies and their emotions.

STAGE FOUR: DEPRESSION, REGRET, SORROW.   Clients in this stage often
regret previous choices they have made about their sexual activity or
about reproduction. They may regret having made career choices that
delayed childbearing. They may feel that having practiced birth control during their childbearing years caused them to miss their chance
to get pregnant—that they changed their fate by choosing to use birth
control. Clients in this stage of grief may also feel sad about what they
cannot have, powerless to change their circumstances, and hopeless
about the possibility of ever becoming a parent.

Clients in this stage may also be beginning the process of acceptance. Because feelings of depression, regret, and sorrow are very uncomfortable to experience, clients who allow themselves to feel these
emotions and accept that they are entitled to do so may be starting to
let go of the things they cannot change. We view the acceptance of
these feelings and their expression as our clients' allowing themselves
to experience the full range of emotions associated with grief.

During this stage of grief your clients may feel profound sorrow
and may not be able to participate in child-focused activities or
continue the medical treatment they had previously pursued so vigorously. They may now feel sad around others who are pregnant or
who have biological children, rather than feeling angry as they may
have in the earlier stages of their grief. Your clients may also begin
to let go of their need to reverse their infertility diagnosis and of
their assumption that a pregnancy is the answer to their sorrow.
They may begin making a distinction between letting go of their
need to be biological parents and keeping the part of them that experienced the loss of biological parenting; that is, they are letting go
of the part of them that is resisting the reality or finality of their
losses, while at the same time honoring the part of them that experienced the loss.

STAGE FIVE: ACCEPTANCE AND INTEGRATION.   During this stage, which usually recurs in response to subsequent losses and throughout clients' lives, clients experience integration of the infertility into their identity. They can acknowledge that the infertility has had an impact on—but does not control—their life. They see the losses as a part of their life experience and have been able to grow from those experiences. Acceptance does not mean an absence of sorrow or disappointment; it means that clients have accepted the infertility as one part of what makes them who they are, and they are not resisting its influence on their life.

Clients in this stage may begin to pursue alternatives to biological parenting because they want to experience parenting and are less concerned with parenting a biological child than they are with parenting a child. They may decide to remain child-free because they have concluded that they have or can have meaning in their lives without experiencing parenting.

Clients may reenter any of these stages of grief when faced with a subsequent loss, such as a miscarried pregnancy or a disrupted adoption. Clients may repeatedly enter and exit various stages of grief, but cycles of grieving are not the same as getting stuck somewhere in the process of grieving.

Acknowledging the Importance of Grieving

Some clients are not able to move through their grief and will instead get stuck at some point in the process. Stagnation in the grief process warrants additional intervention because it severely impairs the client's functioning in all aspects of her life. It can delay our client's reemergence into the broader culture with a newly defined sense of who she is. Ultimately, it prohibits clients from realizing their full potential as human beings.

For some clients, it is much more comfortable to wallow in the emotional expressions of grief—anger, fear, despair, guilt, and the like—than it is to confront, experience, and accept these feelings as part of healing. It is as though holding onto the grief keeps the person connected to the imagined child. Although this is a normal part of grief, it becomes problematic when clients continually reject moving forward in favor of remaining in denial. We have known a few couples who have been stagnant for decades. They have symbolically adopted infertility as a constant companion of the marriage. Without the couple's grief, these marriages have no identity.

Regardless of which phase of grief a client remains stuck in, the reason for the perpetual stagnation is clear: clients fear moving through grief because they unconsciously know that accommodating the loss of the biological child is synonymous with letting go of the dream of biological parenting. Letting go of the dream of biological parenting demands a renegotiation of the client's identity, goals, and tasks in order to move toward a newly defined future. Whether clients are able to respond to these demands or not, on some level many clients sense that working through grief is an intense, draining process.

Therapists can facilitate this process by providing support, guidance, and patience. We consider a client to have accomplished this phase of his grief work (accommodating the loss of the biological child) when he has incorporated his experience of lost fertility and what it represents into his new sense of himself and the meaning his life will have without biological children. Only by taking responsibility for their own healing can clients shed their disenchantment with life as they see it and embrace life for all it can be.

WORKING THROUGH SPECIFIC REPRODUCTIVE LOSSES

In the earlier section on cultural attitudes, we discussed the expectation that all humans will participate in reproduction, which implies that every human being has a responsibility for the continuation of the human race. Regardless of whether or not an individual ascribes to this cultural expectation, a diagnosis of infertility will have implications for that person. One of the most significant implications is the loss of the potential biological child.

We also discussed how the loss of the potential biological child includes the loss of pregnancy, childbirth, participation in the rituals and celebrations surrounding childbirth, and the continuation of the biological family line. As with other infertility-related losses, the loss of a potential biological child may also elicit feelings of depression, inadequacy, anger, and shock. The loss of the potential biological child is also the loss of anticipated opportunities.

Because infertility has a variety of causes, the loss of the potential biological child can occur in different ways. For example, people may lose their potential biological child because they are unable to conceive due to hysterectomy, primary infertility, secondary infertility, or for a variety of diagnosed and undiagnosed male or female malfunctioning reproductive systems. We categorize these losses as *pre-conception losses.* The loss of the potential biological child can also occur after conception through stillbirth and miscarriage. We categorize these losses as *post-conception losses.*

Pre-Conception Losses

The central feature of the loss of a child prior to conception is that the loss is intangible: there is no actual person to grieve, miss, or memorialize. Clients who experience pre-conception losses also are grieving the loss of the opportunity to experience pregnancy and childbirth. Our clients' experiences with pre-conception losses are often made more difficult by the rigors of infertility treatment. Because our clients are often engaged in the process of medical treatment at the same time as they are experiencing pre-conception losses, the time and energy demands of medical treatment often take precedence over working through their grief. In the following sections we define pre-conception losses, discuss the unique features of each loss, and offer treatment strategies for facilitating the grief process of clients who are experiencing these losses.

PRIMARY INFERTILITY.   Clients who experience infertility on their first attempts (thus the term *primary infertility*) to have a biological child are frustrated because they are told not to be concerned until at least one year has passed without conception (according to the medical textbook definition of infertility).

Therefore, unless an obvious problem exists, such as lack of menses or impotency, clients usually begin to educate themselves about their bodies *before* they have received guidance from their physicians. By the time most women visit their gynecologists about their concerns, they may already know about their basal body temperatures, whether or not they are ovulating, and the optimal time for conception. Clients often become very driven to diagnose and fix the problem so that they can get on with the business of conceiving.

Some clients have a diagnosed reason for their infertility; others do not. We believe that knowing (or not knowing) why conception is not occurring affects how the client copes with this situation. When there is a definitive diagnosis, treatments can target the specific problem, and clients can focus on the decision-making process. In addition, there are only so many appropriate treatments to attempt and only so long the treatment can be endured (emotionally, financially, and physically).

When a diagnosis cannot be made about the cause of infertility, treatment proceeds along a continuum, beginning with the least invasive procedures. For example, physicians might recommend that men wear boxer shorts and women chart their basal temperatures. When the simpler interventions fail to produce a viable pregnancy, treatment strategies become more complex. Having undiagnosed infertility can be very frustrating for our clients. It is human nature to want to know why things are not working, and without a logical explanation for the infertility, clients may feel both powerless and without direction. Believing that they have no power or direction makes it difficult for clients to make decisions they feel good about regarding the course and duration of their treatment.

SECONDARY INFERTILITY. *Secondary infertility* describes the condition of being unable to procreate when procreation has been successful in the past. Understandably, clients who already have a biological child (or children) are truly bewildered when they are unable to procreate again. Clients experiencing secondary infertility often express a sense of having failed to accomplish something they were once able to accomplish, as though their prior "success" was completely under their control. These clients also may experience guilt for wanting more than what they have; their guilt sometimes leads them to believe that their friends and family members may view their unceasing efforts to get pregnant again as a lack of appreciation for the biological child they already have.

Clients may also begin to feel that friends and family offer little support and compassion during their battle with secondary infertility. Whether the lack of support is real or imagined, and whether their guilt is appropriate or not, clients with secondary infertility struggle with their desire to continue building their family biologically. It is our role to support them in their efforts to build their families through the means that they believe are most comfortable and appropriate.

We provide this support because whether primary or secondary, infertility is infertility. It is not up to us to compare losses and assume that clients who are experiencing secondary infertility are experiencing grief that is any less intense or valid than clients who are experiencing primary infertility, simply because they already have a child.

Loss is not defined by what one already has but by what one does not have and deeply longs for.

HYSTERECTOMY.   A hysterectomy is the surgical removal of all or part of the uterus. In the past, a hysterectomy would have definitively robbed a woman of her dream to parent a biological child. Since the advances in reproductive technology, however, the only thing that hysterectomy surely denies a woman is the opportunity to experience a pregnancy and childbirth. The distinction between *having* a child and *carrying* a child is significant for the client who dreams of being a biological parent. Whereas some clients who have undergone hysterectomies view their condition as cause to explore child-free living or adoptive parenting, other clients embrace the possibilities available to them through the newest assisted reproductive technology.

Some clients have told us that they favor the "old days," when a hysterectomy meant ending the pursuit for a biological child. These clients prefer having closure forced on them in order to regain some normality in their lives. Because it is now technically possible for women who have undergone hysterectomies to procreate (through egg freezing and surrogacy), closure around the treatment process has become ambiguous. Some clients refer to themselves as infertility treatment "junkies" who continue to pursue their dream of biological parenting, despite the low odds for success.

Facilitating Grief for Pre-Conception Losses

As we said earlier, the central feature of the loss of a child prior to conception is that the loss is intangible: there is only a dream, intricately imagined, that does not fade even when the person awakens to the reality that the dream of biological parenting may not come true. Though very vivid for the client, the dream is difficult to convey to others because of the very nature of dreams.

VERBALIZING LOSSES.   Because pre-conception losses are intangible, it is very difficult for clients to verbalize and legitimize for themselves, let alone to their spouse and therapist, the depth of their suffering. When we work with clients who have experienced pre-conception losses, we try to help them express abstract or intangible losses in concrete terms.

For instance, when one client remarked that she "refused to whine to anyone about a dream that did not come true" lest she be thought of as immature and weak, we asked her to tell us what she had been dreaming of.

> I have been dreaming of having a child with my husband since the day he asked me to marry him. I want so much for the two of us to share the experience of parenting a child. I want to be able to feel a child moving inside of me and to experience the miracle of giving birth. I want to share that experience with my husband. I know we have a lot to offer and that our lives would be enriched by parenting a child. I guess I also want to feel like I have a choice and to stop feeling like there is something wrong with me. Not my body, but me.

After our client expressed these feelings, we talked to her about how clearly she had expressed what she had lost and told her that her explanation seemed neither weak nor immature, but genuine and understandable. We also talked about the concrete losses she had described: the loss of the shared experience of parenting, the loss of the experience of pregnancy and childbirth, the loss of choices, and the loss of her sense of wholeness. These are tangible losses, losses that are worthy of grieving simply because our client was experiencing them. Acknowledging their worth was easier for her when she was able to define clearly what she felt she had lost.

USING BASIC SKILLS. We were able to help this client express her intangible losses in concrete terms because, first, we validated that her dreams were important by asking her to share them with us; second, we empathized with her feelings of loss by expressing our perspective that her feelings seemed genuine and understandable; third, we reframed her explanation of what she had been dreaming of into a list of specifically defined losses. These basic skills can be very effective in facilitating grieving.

DEALING WITH FEELINGS OF SORROW AND INADEQUACY. In our work with clients who have experienced primary infertility or who have had a hysterectomy, we have learned that whether the cause of their infertility is diagnosed or not, they often experience great sorrow over the inability to reproduce. One couple described their inability to conceive as an inability "even to get out of the starting gate." They went on to say that they felt somehow "passed over as contenders in the most important game in life." "After all," they reasoned, "if we cannot perpetuate our own species, how is our contribution to humankind measured?"

We respond to these comments in the same way we respond to all of the perspectives expressed by our clients. We acknowledge their sorrow *first*. As we discussed in Chapter Two, clients will be unable to accept prompts to explore different points of view until they know they have been heard. When they know you have heard them, your clients will begin to ask questions of you that will demonstrate their openness, such as "What do you think?" or "What should we do?" At this point you can respond with your own questions: "Is having a biological child the only contribution you can make to humankind?" "Are there other important games in life besides the parenting game?"

Be prepared to provide sample answers to your clients who may have no response to your questions. For instance, you can name well-known people who never had biological children, who have made significant contributions to humankind, such as Jesus, Helen Keller, Tennessee Williams, Mother Teresa, and Tom Cruise. You can then ask your clients to consider individuals whom they know personally that fit this same category.

You can also explore other important "games" people play in life besides the parenting game, such as the professional, partnership, altruistic, and creative games. Developing this self-awareness is challenging for clients experiencing infertility, because not realizing the dream of biological parenting confuses clients' sense of who they are and what their lives are about. As you help clients who are experiencing primary infertility to explore other ways in which they can feel included, you help them understand their own identities.

ACKNOWLEDGING LOSSES OF SECONDARY INFERTILITY.   As we explained earlier, loss is not defined by what one already has but by what one does not have and deeply longs for. We always keep this in mind when we work with clients who are experiencing secondary infertility. This distinction came to light for us with Anne, a client who had five biological children and was unable to get pregnant again. She told us,

> I came from a traditional Catholic family. There were ten children. My husband, Joe, is also Catholic and one of eleven children. We dreamed of having a large family like the ones we came from, and consider our-

selves to be halfway there. Don't get me wrong. It is not as though we do not love the children we do have, or that they are somehow not enough. It is we who do not feel like we are enough. Like we have somehow failed in our attempts to create what we thought was the perfect family.

Before Anne and her husband pursued infertility treatment, we explored other ways to define the "perfect family." Both Anne and Joe came to understand that they had always defined *perfect* with a number rather than by valuing the uniqueness of each member or the path by which each person came to the family. Anne and Joe walked away from their one and only session realizing that they—not (what they thought were) the mandates of their religion—were responsible for defining *perfect*.

With Anne and Joe, as with all clients experiencing secondary infertility, we paid great attention to the effect their sorrow had on the parenting of the children already in the home. Some clients express resentment toward their biological child(ren) for not being the child(ren) they dream of having. These clients seem both to take for granted what they have and to glamorize what they are missing. This reaction is damaging to the entire family unit, and usually manifests as bottled-up emotions expressed at inappropriate times and in inappropriate ways.

Thus, we need to encourage clients to grieve for the lost biological child. Once they are able to experience the full range of emotions associated with their loss, they are able to accept their predicament. Acceptance replaces the old reactive behavior with proactive behavior. Ultimately, clients gain a new perspective that enables them to see that their existing child(ren) have nothing to do with the imagined child. Having made this distinction, clients are able to enjoy parenting the child(ren) they have, while pursuing infertility treatment as a separate endeavor. In addition, clients who are able authentically and appropriately to express their emotions throughout the course of infertility treatment will serve as healthy role models for their biological child(ren).

Post-Conception Losses

The central feature of the loss of a child after a pregnancy is that the expectant parents have begun to bond with a specific child. And as the pregnancy progresses, so does the bonding. Achieved pregnancies, even in the midst of an infertility battle, also are viewed as successes that give expecting parents hope for fulfilling the longed-for dream of parenting. When that hope is shattered, the loss is usually sudden and unexpected.

Expectant parents may have already tried to determine the moment of their child's conception and the actual month of their child's birth and birthday. They may know the child's gender and may have already chosen a name, prepared a nursery, purchased clothing and supplies, and started referring to themselves as Mom and Dad. Clearly, clients who experience the loss of a child after a pregnancy has actually taken place face issues that seriously complicate the grieving process. In the next sections we discuss the impact of losing a child through stillbirth or miscarriage, discuss the unique features of each loss, and offer treatment strategies for facilitating the grief process associated with post-conception losses.

STILLBIRTH.   Stillbirth is the birth of a dead baby. Losing a child that has been healthy throughout a pregnancy is an exceptionally difficult reproductive loss to endure. The baby who is dead upon delivery was, in fact, a vital, active being with whom the expectant parents had an intimate relationship. Expectant parents are anxious to meet the person who has been gently maneuvering inside its mother's body for so long, the person they have caressed, sung to, and carried lovingly with eager anticipation.

The reality of the life inside is often compounded by ultrasound photographs and the knowledge of the baby's gender through amniocentesis. For nine months, the expectant mother literally eats and breathes for her unborn child and is always conscious of her responsibility to provide a healthy environment for her baby. In addition to keeping the temporary "home" healthy for the developing baby, the parents often rearrange and prepare the house for the baby they are expecting. Clients have told us that nothing is more torturous than coming home from the hospital and confronting the cheery nursery that was intended for the baby who has been left behind. The nursery door is often closed indefinitely, and the actual room becomes a never-used space. It becomes a painful reminder of all that was hoped for and lost.

Unlike other lost imagined children, stillbirths carry the multiple burdens of managing labor and delivery; funerals or memorial services; religious rituals; the return or storage of baby gifts; return of the mother's body to normal; and the holding, seeing, and naming of the baby who has died. Although the baby has never come home and been newly integrated into the family's routines and lifestyle, these burdens make it seem as though the baby had a life outside the womb. Parents of stillborn babies typically experience all the normal grief reactions experienced by anyone who loses someone he or she has deeply loved.

MISCARRIAGE.   In a miscarriage, the embryo or fetus is expelled from the uterus before it is sufficiently developed to survive. By definition, miscarriage includes both first trimester embryos and second trimester fetuses, as well as tubal pregnancies that rupture or dislodge before detection for surgical removal. Most commonly, however, miscarriages occur during the first trimester when the pregnancy has yet to become visible to others.

Expectant parents often delay sharing the news of their pregnancy until after the first trimester is behind them. Many parents, both those with and without a history of fertility problems, often "wait and see" how the pregnancy is faring before telling others. Many parents view delaying the news of their pregnancy as a way to protect themselves from having to face people should the pregnancy be unsuccessful. This view is particularly common for parents who have experienced multiple miscarriages. Not having to face people with unfortunate news may seem like a relief to grieving parents in the wake of a miscarriage, but we believe that silence can complicate the grieving process. Henry and Carrie illustrate this point:

CARRIE: After the second miscarriage, I just could not bear to see the faces of everyone we had told. It was so painful that I swore if we got pregnant again, no one would know about it until our baby was born!

HENRY: Then, we got pregnant again. And I was all for keeping the news a secret. So we did.

THERAPIST: And what happened when you miscarried again?

CARRIE: We had nowhere to go but to each other.

THERAPIST: Were you not able to support one another?

CARRIE: Yes, we were. But we needed more. I needed my girlfriends, and Henry needed to talk to friends, too.

HENRY: Boy, was that a surprise. I started noticing that I slammed a lot of stuff around. I was always in a hurry, and got ticked-off easily.

THERAPIST: Were those unusual behaviors for you?

HENRY: Really, yes. I am a pretty easy-going guy.

CARRIE: That is true.

THERAPIST: So what do you think was going on?

HENRY: I think I felt like a caged animal. Only what I did not know was that I was the cage for my own self. Do you know what I mean?

THERAPIST: I am not sure. Explain it to me another way.

HENRY: I wanted to let my anger and disappointment burst out of myself. Keeping our miscarriage a secret from everyone made me want to burst. I just could not hold it in anymore.

THERAPIST: So what did you do?

CARRIE: About two months later, we agreed to talk to our friends and family.

THERAPIST: Did it help?

CARRIE: Definitely. As soon as we started talking, it took us back to the moment we lost the baby. It was almost like keeping the secret had stopped us in time.

Even though friends and family probably want to know what is happening, we are not suggesting that grieving parents share their news for the sake of informing people who care about them. What we are suggesting is that through opening up, through facing and accepting their loss, grieving parents will be further along on their healing journey.

Facilitating Grief for Post-Conception Losses

Clients who experience losing a baby through stillbirth or miscarriage experience varying degrees of posttraumatic stress and deserve to work with a therapist who fully understands the features of this disorder. (For a complete discussion of Posttraumatic Stress Disorder and infertility, see Chapter Four.) Posttraumatic stress is one critical issue that complicates the grieving process for these clients. Another is the very nature of the parent-child relationship.

LOSS OF THE PARENT-CHILD RELATIONSHIP.   This is the only human relationship in which one person is innately dependent on the other for survival, for a designated period of time. The majority of pregnancies are nurtured by extensive prenatal care, carried to term, and delivered without incident. Once outside the womb, babies rely on their parents to meet their basic needs for survival through the provision of love and attention, food, clothing, and shelter. Even after children grow up and assert their independence, and throughout their adulthood, *parents feel responsible for their children's well-being.* Parents blame themselves when things don't go well, and they are full of pride when they do. Even psychologically healthy parents, who have been able to let go of their adult children and trust in their children's ability to care for themselves, wonder if they could not have been even more effective as a parent and have made better choices.

In abnormal situations, when babies in utero do not survive, parents are at risk for feeling as though they have failed their children at the most basic level. Thus, when stillbirths and miscarriages occur, grieving may be complicated by the parents' sense that they are somehow responsible for the loss of their baby. As a therapist, you must understand that there are no magic words that will alleviate your clients' guilt. Furthermore, there is a strong possibility, even with time, growth, and perspective, that a shadow of guilt will always be with your clients. Therefore, you must facilitate your clients' acceptance of their reactions to the loss, just as you help them strive to accept infertility and the aftermath of stillbirth and miscarriage.

CULTURALLY ACKNOWLEDGED LOSSES.   When parents are grieving the loss of a stillborn child, they are supported because their loss is socially sanctioned. This loss is recognized by the broader culture because the reality of the baby was visible throughout its mother's pregnancy. The stillborn child was expected, nurtured, and planned for in the parents' lives. When the news of the baby's death is conveyed to everyone who knew of the pregnancy, compassion and sympathy abound, and support is available. This support can be a key factor in the healing of the grieving parents. Parents who feel forced to grieve in isolation because their loss is not socially acknowledged lose this avenue of support.

CULTURALLY MISUNDERSTOOD LOSSES.   When clients experience a miscarriage, their grief is more difficult to convey and to understand fully. Our clients tell us that many people respond to the news of a miscarriage by saying things like "Well, at least you're still young and can try again" and "Maybe it's better that it happened now and not later when you would have been more attached to the baby." Although comments like these may be intended to help our clients move on, they fail to acknowledge the loss that the grieving parents have experienced. And we have learned that a lack of acknowledgment is painful and does not facilitate additional expressions of grief.

As we discussed at length in Chapter One, when people can express what it is that pains them so deeply, they can heal. Grieving parents will undoubtedly want to share their shattered dream of the parenting experience, the loss of the pregnancy symptoms, and the frustration in having come so close and yet still ending up without a baby. However, when grieving parents share their grief with others who are not able to acknowledge their loss, they may wind up feeling misunderstood, frustrated, and uncomfortable.

We therefore encourage our clients to choose carefully those with whom they will share their grief. We acknowledge that not all of the people who may ask about the miscarriage will be those with whom our clients will want to share their feelings. But sharing these issues with a few appropriate individuals will mean that parents do not have to grieve alone, in spite of the lack of prescribed rituals for miscarriage in our culture.

We also encourage clients to explore their grief and the meaning of their losses in a more solitary manner. One way they can do this is through writing a journal.

EXPLORING GRIEF THROUGH JOURNAL WRITING.   When we assign journal writing to clients, we know that many people are not adept at expressing themselves through writing and need specific guidelines when beginning their journals. We explain to our clients that journal writing is helpful for several reasons: it provides them with an opportunity to examine their thoughts, ideas, and feelings; it helps them gain self-understanding and insight into themselves; and it helps them discuss the things that are important to them and explore emotions they may not have been aware of until they see them in writing.

Journal writing is also a creative process that facilitates healing. Clients can use a journal as a platform for creating a relationship with the self that develops self-love, self-awareness, and self-esteem. It can also be a platform to develop relationships with others through unsent letters and unspoken dialogues. Journal writing is particularly helpful for our clients because the experience of infertility can threaten them at the core of their identity. These clients can rediscover themselves as the individuals they believed themselves to be prior to their diagnosis.

—∿∿—

Whether clients experience their reproductive losses as a failure to meet cultural expectations or as a rude awakening to the end of a longed-for dream, all are challenged to integrate these reproductive losses into their identity. Meeting this challenge is a process, and as the chapter's opening epigraph implies, there is a specific manner by which self-discovery occurs. The client's journey toward integration usually begins with the search for understanding about how infertility influences his future, goals, and self-acceptance. In Chapter Six we explore the implications of infertility on our clients' sexuality and discuss treatment strategies for working with clients when they are experiencing difficulty with these issues.

Dealing with Sexuality and Infertility

The first step toward self-esteem for most of us is not to learn but to unlearn. We need to demystify the forces that have told us what we should be before we can value what we are.

—*Gloria Steinem,* Revolution from Within

Regardless of how religion, parents, society, schools, and experiences shape sexual views, human beings are undeniably sexual beings with drives for both pleasure and procreation. If we lived in an ideal world, both male and female children would be allowed to discover their emerging sexuality in a context of support and enthusiasm. Their questions would be met with truths, freedom, and patience. As they traveled through adolescence, children would seek peer support and explore appropriate avenues for healthy sexual expression. As adults, men and women could enter into sexual relationships with a clear sense of who they are and what they could realistically contribute in their interactions.

In addition, educational curricula would provide specific information on *all* matters related to sex and sexuality. Beginning in elementary school, children would learn about reproduction: how it occurs, and why in some cases it may not. Secondary schools would provide direct information about sexually transmitted diseases, how to prevent premature pregnancy, and how to cope with increased sexual drives. This kind of candid, factual exposure to sexuality and related issues, *at an early age,* would better prepare the individual who receives a diagnosis of infertility. The individual would, at the very least, know that infertility is a possible diagnosis for some people.

In an ideal world, children would grow up with parents who are themselves healthy sexual beings. Parents would speak openly and clearly to their children. No one would be slapped for touching themselves, and no one would be hushed for speaking about genitalia. No one would experience their sexuality in the context of violence or violation. In a perfect world, people would genuinely know themselves and possess the maturity to allow both their masculine and feminine aspects free expression. Our culture would sanction the discussion of sexuality through intimacy and genuine interaction, rather than through humor and vulgarity. We imagine this perfect world easily because it is the polar opposite of how we truly live. Receiving a diagnosis of infertility in this real world is like having insult added to injury.

Although sexuality is a basic component of the human identity, it is the cause of much confusion and embarrassment. It is often denied, repressed, and misunderstood. People seem to separate themselves from their sexuality with respect to drive and pleasure, yet comfortably acknowledge their sexuality with respect to the basic function of procreation. When a client receives a diagnosis of infertility, the comfortably acknowledged purpose of sexuality vanishes and creates a void that jeopardizes basic functioning. The client is suddenly left with a host of disturbing questions that have no clear answers: "What is wrong with me? Are we not *doing it* right? What is God's plan for me?" The experience of infertility is difficult to integrate into healthy sexuality.

Although some of the changes that your clients will experience in their sexuality will be directly related to sexual functioning (for example, difficulty with becoming sexually aroused, maintaining an erection, being able to have an orgasm, or experiencing sexual pleasure), a detailed discussion of these issues is beyond the scope of this book. There are many excellent resources written by professionals who specialize in sexual dysfunction that are available for those who want to learn more about these issues and how to treat them in the therapeutic setting. (One of the books we recommend and frequently consult on behalf of our clients is *Night Thoughts: Reflections of a Sex Therapist,* by Avodah K. Offit.)

This chapter addresses the impact of infertility on sexuality, acknowledging that for most humans, sexuality, even without the impact of infertility, is an *already compromised realm of functioning*. We also address the impact of infertility on the sexual relationship and discuss how clients can experience healthy sexuality despite a diagnosis of infertility. We have included two detailed cases in this chapter because the issue of sexuality and infertility is complex, and healthy sexuality after a diagnosis of infertility requires the reintegration of our clients' psychosocial, sexual, and biological identities. The case histories detail two couples' experiences with their sexuality after a diagnosis of infertility; their stories demonstrate the multiple challenges that your clients will face in their efforts to sustain healthy sexual relationships.

UNDERSTANDING BARRIERS TO HEALTHY SEXUALITY

The development of healthy sexuality is impeded by society's influence on the definition of appropriate sexual expression and by the influence of the roles that men and women play in procreation. In order to understand fully the impact that a diagnosis of infertility can have on our clients' sexuality, we must first understand the context in which sexuality is developed.

Influence of Society

Unfortunately, the society in which we live stifles the expression of human sexuality. Many people pretend they have no sex drive, and those who do acknowledge their desires are criticized and disdained. Our culture dictates who and what people *should* be, and does not support who people really *are*. Ironically, people refuse to listen to themselves, even as their deepest selves shout for liberation and natural expression. This is what makes a diagnosis of infertility so hard to bear: How can clients express their frustrations with infertility in a culture that does not allow free expression of their sexuality under *normal* circumstances?

You probably are familiar with the 1950s children's book series about the adventurous little monkey who was always getting into trouble. The monkey, who represented children, was introduced in all of the stories as good, but curious. The implication in all the tales is that if he could just stop being curious, then everything would be all right. Replacing the word *but* with the word *and*—good, and curious— would lead us to the ideal world in which the monkey's goodness is genuinely rather than conditionally accepted. Unfortunately, the perspective that curiosity is a character defect is all too common in our society. This judgmental perspective is found in such well-known clichés as "Children should be seen and not heard," "Don't speak unless spoken to," and "Curiosity killed the cat." All of these clichés are designed to stifle a child's natural self-expression. Children learn from an early age an entire repertoire of "don'ts." If they are compliant, they are considered well behaved. As adults, they are deemed mature and civilized. We assert that what they really become is repressed, frustrated, and confused. Because people are socially directed to deny self-expression, it is no mystery that human beings are dysfunctional at a most *basic* level of self-expression: sexuality.

Influence of Roles in Procreation

Everything that *is* known about sexuality is communicated to individuals from the moment parents learn of their child's gender. Whether it is determined in utero or in the delivery room, gender automatically tells parents which colors to paint the nursery, which toys to buy, and which vocal tones with which to speak. All these gender-related variables contribute to the ways in which individuals ultimately express their sexuality. Children observe parents' dressing habits, body language, and communication style. And as they grow older, individuals are expected to model their same-sex parent.

Because all human beings have a mother and a father, it is reasonable to assert that everyone has opinions about the role definitions of mothers and fathers. Of course, it can be a rude awakening to realize that parents, first and foremost, are human beings. But whether individuals model or reject these roles in their lives, people nonetheless integrate the meaning of these roles into their sexuality. This integration into our sexuality of our ideas of what it means to be a mother or father is a powerful phenomenon, because underlying the integration is the assumption that the individual, too, will be a mother or a father. How often have you heard "I want to be just like my mom" or "I hope to be nothing like my dad"? What these statements demonstrate is that sexuality is fundamentally influenced by our belief that we epitomize masculinity and femininity through the function of procreating rather than through our interpretation of what it is to be a human being.

The problem with the assumption that one will become a mother or a father is that many people will *not* become parents. In effect, this assumption creates the possibility of failure for numerous adults. For instance, some individuals reach adulthood and for a number of reasons decide not to marry or not to have children. Although they try to honor their true selves, the messages they hear from inside and outside themselves force them to question their sexuality from the very core. Would a *real* woman choose not to be a mother? Would a *real* man be unable or choose not to impregnate his wife? Our society has people believing that if they are the epitome of the prescribed definitions of masculinity or femininity, then they will live happily ever after. So what happens when the ability to procreate is threatened or denied? It seriously affects a person's ability to express their sexuality.

THE INFLUENCE OF INFERTILITY ON SEXUAL RELATIONSHIPS

Infertility can have a direct influence on a client's identity as a sexual being, and many clients who are experiencing infertility will therefore also experience changes in their sexual relationships. The primary changes in sexuality that our clients have reported are that infertility affects intimacy, compromises privacy, and creates pressure to conceive.

Affects Intimacy

The obvious connections between the act of sex and reproduction strongly influence the relationship between sexuality and infertility. However, sexuality is not limited to the act of sex. Sexuality certainly includes the physical aspects of sex, but it also includes attitudes about sexual expression (expressions of gender identity, and sexual preferences, behaviors, and needs) and perceptions about biological roles in reproduction.

When our clients' efforts to conceive a child repeatedly fail, the association between sex and the failure to conceive may begin to influence every sexual encounter. When clients are affected this way, sex may no longer be a spontaneous activity that they share to express themselves and their feelings; sex instead becomes a part of the predictable cycle of false hope and disappointment. Although the association between sex and feelings of failure may not always be overwhelming, or even prohibitive, it is ever present.

When our clients begin to feel as if their sexual relationship represents their failure to conceive, one or both of the partners may begin to question their ability to "properly" function where sex is concerned. For many clients it then becomes difficult to determine whether the infertility led to problems in the sexual relationship or problems in the sexual relationship led to the infertility. For example, clients may begin to wonder whether the infertility is correlated with their adequacy as a sexual partner, with the frequency and timing of sexual activity with their partner, or with the level of stress in their lives and its impact on their attitude toward their sexual relationship. Furthermore, when our clients receive advice about their fertility problems, this advice often includes such meaningless suggestions as "Just relax" or "Maybe you're trying too hard." Thus, both the absence of a pregnancy and the attitudes and comments of others reinforce our clients' concerns about the causal relationship between their ability to function sexually and the infertility. With this kind of external and internal pressure, a once comfortable sexual relationship may begin to suffer; an already difficult one goes from bad to worse.

Compromises Privacy

In our culture, sexuality is private, often obsessively so. Sexuality also is regularly misconstrued as the sole barometer of the success of our romantic relationships (a satisfactory sex life indicates that our relationships are healthy). On the contrary, our practice has taught us that open communication and frank discussion of sexuality are far better barometers of a successful relationship. Unfortunately, discussion of sexuality is typically not encouraged during our formative years, and most of our clients are not comfortable discussing their sexuality in a professional setting. When infertility forces people to discuss their sex lives with their partners and their physicians, the compulsory nature of the discussion minimizes its benefits.

As we discussed in Chapter Three, medical treatment for infertility takes our clients' sexuality out of their home and into the laboratory. Tests are administered, samples given, temperatures charted, eggs harvested, and medications taken. The physician and his or her staff become expert advisers on a couple's most private relationship. When medical professionals become a part of a couple's sexual relationship, it can disconnect our clients from their sexuality, an intensely personal element of their being. Someone who hasn't experienced this process may find it easy to minimize the disassociation that occurs. This situation is an extreme form of what a woman endures in the gynecologist's stirrups: a part of her person that in all other circumstances is kept private is now the focus of intrusive attention and is simultaneously curtained off from her view. Thus the alienation is both literal and symbolic.

In addition to feeling that their privacy has been invaded, couples may feel that they must have "sex on demand." When the calendar dictates that the fertile period has arrived, it doesn't matter whether one or both partners has had a bad day at work, one of them is sick, or their parents are visiting—when it's time to have sex, it's time to have sex. As if that were not bad enough, the couple must also report to their physician about the frequency and timing of their sexual encounters during the "fertile" period.

Creates Pressure to Conceive

As the length of treatment increases and the medical options for achieving a pregnancy diminish, your clients may experience an increased sense of urgency in their desire to have a child. As their sense of immediacy increases, so will the pressure for sexual activity to result in a pregnancy. As our clients struggle to have a child, their sexual relationship may take on new meaning. Where sex may once have been about physical pleasure, the manifestation of intimacy, and the physical expression of emotions, it now includes the goal of pregnancy. Infertility often prevents our clients from achieving the goal of pregnancy, and thus one of the needs in the sexual relationship remains unmet. If our clients' sexual encounters continually result in even mild disappointment, it is likely that the sexual relationship will begin to deteriorate.

Biology imposes time constraints that apply even more pressure for sexual activity to result in pregnancy. As people age, their fertility naturally decreases. This decrease is especially pronounced in women over thirty-five. Couples experiencing infertility may feel that they are in a race against time that they cannot win. Oftentimes unknowing friends and family exacerbate couples' feelings of despair by pointing out the very things that couples fear the most.

For example, after a very stressful experience at Joy's parents house over Thanksgiving, Joy and her husband, Adam, made the difficult decision to stay at home for the December holidays. Adam described the Thanksgiving visit as "four days of 'We don't understand what you're waiting for. If you don't get with the program you're going to be too old to enjoy the kids once you have them.'" Although Adam and Joy knew that her parents did not mean any harm and that their families would be disappointed about their decision, they both agreed that they could not endure another holiday like the last one.

Both internally and externally applied pressure for sexual activity to result in a pregnancy can have detrimental effects on our clients' sexuality. For instance, clients may feel that the expression of their sexuality has become secondary to achieving a pregnancy or that the failure to achieve a pregnancy symbolizes their failure as a male or female because they have not fulfilled their biological roles in reproduction. These feelings of failure and inadequacy are not consistent with a healthy sexual relationship or a healthy sexual identity.

THE STORY OF DEAN AND RACHEL

Because it is common for clients to be disturbed and frightened by the changes in their sexuality, we present a case that illustrates what happens when clients experience turbulence in their sexuality after a diagnosis of infertility. This case includes some of this couple's psychosocial history because we have found that background information is essential to our understanding of the impact that infertility has had on our clients.

You can solicit background information during an interview, or you can ask your clients to complete an autobiography. (Autobiography guidelines are included in Chapter Eleven.) The autobiography is designed to obtain information on clients' family of origin; their educational, work, and relationship or marital history; their religious views; and their hobbies and interests. We also use autobiographies to help clients clarify their values and their perception of themselves, their family, and their spouse, and to help clients explore the various roles they have played and still play in their life. It is also used to help clients identify and explore past and present events that have had an impact on their life. As you know, it is difficult to understand how your clients have gotten to where they are if you do not know anything about the paths that have led them there.

Psychosocial History

We originally introduced you to Rachel and Dean in Chapter Three. They shared a traditional marriage and had been married for eight and a half years. Rachel was thirty-four years old, Dean was thirty-seven.

Rachel had three brothers and one sister. All of her siblings were married and had biological children. Dean had one sister who was also married and had three biological daughters. Dean was a business professional and owned a consulting firm. He worked a sixty-hour week ten miles from his home. Rachel stopped working as an administrative assistant when she married, and had always prided herself on her ability to provide her husband (and future children) with a beautiful, well-managed home.

For the first five years of their marriage, Rachel and Dean had used birth control as they "settled into" life together. They had always assumed that they would have children. Two years before we began seeing the couple, after one year of trying to get pregnant, Dean was diagnosed as having a low sperm count with low motility. Rachel had no diagnosable barriers to reproduction. It had always been important to Dean, as the only heir to his family's name, that he have a son to whom to leave his business and his name. They had been struggling to conceive for three years. So far, treatment had not affected the count or motility of Dean's sperm, and five intrauterine insemination attempts had failed. Dean's insurance company had paid for the first three procedures, but the couple had incurred the cost of the last two treatments. The couple had committed to one more procedure before considering alternatives to biological parenting.

When Dean and Rachel inquired about adoption at a local agency, Dean made it clear that he would only consider adopting a girl because he believed that an adopted son could not legitimately carry on the family name. Their adoption worker requested counseling about his preference as a prerequisite to an adoption home study. Dean refused to discuss in counseling his belief that a male child is the only legitimate heir to his name, because he knew that this opinion would not change. Rachel reported that she grew sadder by the day as her purpose in the marriage and her role as expectant mother seemed further from her grasp.

Impact on the Relationship

Rachel had spent the last three years of her life planning for and "waiting" for a baby. In the meantime, Dean had gradually increased the number of hours he worked during a week. Whereas the weekends had once been considered "sacred" times to be with Rachel, he was working six- to eight-hour days on Saturdays and Sundays. Rachel felt overlooked and unappreciated. She was also angry and sad. Above all, she missed the time spent with her husband and wondered why she was no longer enough for him. Dean continued to say that his long hours had nothing to do with her, but that the business needed attention. Rachel believed that Dean worked more because work was an area in his life that he could influence, whereas he was unable to influence his fertility. In a sense, the business had become Dean's baby, and Rachel was still at home waiting, either for a baby or for Dean.

The tension between Rachel and Dean was at an all-time high. They were not communicating well. They were not taking time to be with one another, and they argued frequently. Dean grew more resentful of the infertility that had taken away his dream to father a son, while Rachel grew more discouraged as she grieved over the loss of her marriage as it once was and the prospective loss of the child she had always imagined mothering.

Rachel wanted Dean to know that she felt he was a real man, whether they had biological children or not. He refused Rachel's efforts to support and comfort him because he considered her gestures to be condescending and provoked by pity. Rachel felt powerless and lost. Dean was frustrated and confused.

Impact on Sexuality

For Rachel and Dean, their sex life had always been an integral part of the marriage. They had never discussed their sex life before the infertility diagnosis. They described their sex life during the first five years of their marriage as fun and spontaneous. They agreed that Dean always initiated sex and Rachel willingly responded.

Shortly after the diagnosis that revealed Dean's condition, he became unable to sustain an erection and ultimately lost the ability to achieve one at all. After a year and a half of trying to overcome the dysfunction on their own, Dean agreed to attend counseling so long as he was not expected to discuss his impotency.

In individual sessions with Rachel, she provided this account of a typical sexual encounter:

> I feel so bad for him, I mean, I don't care if we have sex or not. I'm just
> so happy to have him home, to have him close to me. Lately I've tried
> to be the one to initiate things between us but I get the idea that he
> still wants to be the one to start things up. So I've been trying to do

things that will make him do that. I buy really nice nightwear, and I do my nails just like he likes them, and my hair, too. Sometimes he approaches me and sometimes he doesn't. But when he does, I can just see that he's afraid that it is not going to work out again. And he tries so hard, I wish he would just relax. I feel like I can't try to help him along in any way because he wants to be in control. But then when I do nothing I wonder if he is not somehow blaming me for his not being turned on. Well, he is turned on, it is just that he doesn't respond anymore. And then after that, well, he rolls over and I try to hold him, but I may as well not even be there.

I am so confused. Nothing has ever prepared me for this. I just want him to feel like a man again. I do not understand why this baby thing has shaken him up so much. I mean, we can always adopt. But he has it in his head that it has to be his baby from his body or there isn't any point.

I don't know how much longer we can last like this. Our bedroom used to be a place where we could relax and enjoy each other. Now it just represents such sadness. And I am getting angry because he is being so harsh with himself and it's going to wreck everything. None of the things that used to arouse him work anymore and he flat-out refuses to talk about it. You know, it's real funny. As long as we were having sex on a regular basis, I never thought about what I wanted. But now I feel like I have lost my partner, and I am real aware that I have needs that are not being met. Not just for sex but for closeness. That closeness is what I really miss the most. And the laughter. Sex used to be fun. Now we dread it and really seem to be avoiding it more and more.

Rachel's account of what was happening between her and Dean is common among couples who share traditional roles in their marriage. The male partner takes charge of most decisions, including when and when not to have sex. Not only did Dean initiate sex, but Rachel followed his lead throughout each sexual encounter.

When a diagnosis of infertility, especially one in which the condition is held by the male partner, shifts the way in which couples relate to one another, the entire sexual dynamic is altered. Roles that were never verbally defined or communicated change without warning. In this couple's situation, in which Dean had always initiated sex, Rachel was left with this responsibility. Furthermore, Dean did not usually respond to Rachel's overtures the way Rachel used to respond to Dean.

Couples report that it seems as though they are suddenly in uncharted waters without oars, maps, or compass. They do not know how they ended up in this situation or how to get out of it. What makes this change in sexuality particularly challenging for traditional marriages is that healing requires verbal communication between partners. Open communication enables these couples to consciously redefine the ways in which the partners relate to one another.

We helped Dean and Rachel examine the old ways in which they expressed themselves sexually. This examination included a look at both partners' ideas of what it is to be a man and what it means to be a woman:

THERAPIST: Dean, how do you determine whether you are honoring your role as a man and a husband to Rachel?

DEAN: Well, I bring in all the income. I make sure Rachel has a good time in bed, and I intend to be a father to a son.

THERAPIST: Is there anything else?

DEAN: Yes. I do think I should be the one to initiate lovemaking.

THERAPIST: What do you think of those definitions, Rachel? Do you agree with them?

RACHEL: Oh yes, I always have. Dean is the perfect man.

THERAPIST: So how do you, then, define yourself as a woman and a wife, Rachel?

RACHEL: I am the manager of the home, a willing sexual partner, and hope to be a mother to a child.

THERAPIST: Has your experience with infertility altered those roles?

DEAN: Only in how we are behaving, but not in what we believe.

RACHEL: That is why we are having such a hard time.

Ideally, examining beliefs and roles in sexuality allows for growth in the marital relationship as well as in the sexual relationship. For Dean and Rachel to find one another again, they would have to accept that infertility had had a permanent impact on their lives together. However, it would be possible to redefine their mutual expectations of one another despite their infertility diagnosis. Perhaps Rachel would find ways to express her femaleness through other avenues besides through her home and through her role as an expectant mother. Dean might be able to redefine his role as a man without regard to his ability to procreate or maintain an erection.

Ironically, when couples alleviate the pressure to "perform" in rigidly defined roles, most discover new aspects of each other and themselves that were not visible prior to the infertility diagnosis. Through rediscovering the individuals they are married to, many partners experience their sexuality in ways they never imagined possible. We will revisit the case of Rachel and Dean in Chapter Ten in the Infertility and Identity sessions.

We have seen that infertility can serve as a catalyst for changes in our clients' sexuality. Sexuality may become a function of reproduction instead of reproduction being a function of sexuality. When our clients' sexuality and infertility become inextricably intertwined, we must help our clients clarify the boundaries between their sexual relationship and their desire to have a child, as we did with Dean and Rachael. When clients who are experiencing infertility can make clear distinctions between their sexuality and the infertility, they increase their chances of having a healthy sexual relationship.

EXPERIENCING HEALTHY SEXUALITY

In general, healthy sexuality requires that clients define themselves from a psychosocial as well as a biological perspective. Infertility often leads clients to define themselves solely by the parts they play in reproduction, including defining themselves or their partners according to the biological limitations of the infertility. If each partner, after a diagnosis of infertility, can retain or develop a sense of his of her sexuality that goes beyond biological considerations, the couple may begin to reexperience a sexual relationship that is based on genuine interaction and true self-expression.

When we encounter couples who are struggling to integrate an infertility diagnosis into their sexuality, we ask each client to define all of the things that make him or her male or female, husband or wife, son or daughter, and so on. In other words, we ask our clients to view the infertility as but one aspect of their whole selves. (We often use the integrity wheel exercise in Chapter Eleven to facilitate this discussion.) We emphasize the idea that sexuality involves much more than procreation, and strive to assist couples to define themselves as more than their diagnosis. Our clients can grow tremendously when they cultivate a definition of self that includes the infertility and everything else that makes them who they are.

As we explained earlier in this chapter, our clients have identified three specific ways that infertility influences their sexuality: it affects intimacy, compromises privacy, and creates pressure to conceive. Therefore, our work with clients to help them experience healthy sexuality includes work on reclaiming intimacy, maintaining privacy, and alleviating pressure to conceive.

Reclaiming Intimacy

Partners who have allowed infertility to become the primary focus of their relationship face a major stumbling block in the reclamation of healthy sexuality. The partners may also be basing their future happiness on a pregnancy. Each sexual encounter thus becomes a possible means to an end, namely, conception. This kind of pressure simply is not conducive to a relaxed or spontaneous sexual relationship. In her book *Gift from the Sea,* Anne Morrow Lindbergh offers a perspective that we believe is useful for clients who are struggling to balance their desire for a pregnancy with their sexual relationship. She writes, "One never knows what chance treasures these easy unconscious rollers [waves] may toss up[, but they] . . . must not be sought for or—heaven forbid!—dug for. No, no dredging of the sea-bottom here. That would defeat one's purpose. Patience, patience, patience, is what the sea teaches. Patience and faith. One should lie empty, open, and choiceless as a beach—waiting for a gift from the sea."

As Lindbergh tells us, when we limit our focus to the *outcome* of our actions, we sometimes forget that the action in and of itself can be rewarding. In other words, rather than focusing on a pregnancy as the end result of sexual activity, our clients must learn to be patient and enjoy the journey. When clients remain open to the pleasures of expressing their sexuality, rather than focus on the goal of pregnancy, they are much more likely to remember and experience the many gifts that intimacy and the expression of sexuality have to offer.

Maintaining Privacy

The loss of sexual privacy is an unavoidable part of medical treatment for infertility. However, we can help our clients cope with this loss by encouraging them to rely on one another for support and by facilitating open discussions between partners about sexuality and reproduction. (We must let our clients set the pace of these discussions according to their own levels of comfort.) One of the homework assignments we give couples to help increase their comfort level involves going to a bookstore to select a book about reproduction and sexuality. We instruct each partner to read the same chapter and then privately discuss the contents with each other. The couple then has an opportunity to learn the medical terminology that may have previously been unknown to them and develop the vocabulary to interact on a more clinical level with physicians and other medical professionals. This exercise encourages clients to educate themselves about their own and their partner's body and allows them to do so in an environment of their choosing and at a pace that is comfortable for them.

We also encourage clients to consider carefully the people to whom they choose to disclose the specifics of the infertility and its impact on their sexuality. We do this because our clients have told us that the initial disappointments of infertility frequently prompt them to discuss their condition with anyone who will listen. The result is often tons of advice but very little support. We ask couples to focus on talking to one another and on learning to provide support to each other and then making decisions about sharing information with others. We regularly remind our clients that intimacy depends on privacy, understanding, and respect, and ask them to concentrate on protecting the intimacy in their relationship as an antidote to the "medicalization" of their sexuality.

Alleviating Pressure to Conceive

When our clients are experiencing increasing pressure to conceive, and their sex life seems to be focused solely on the goal of pregnancy, we encourage them to engage in sexual activity that does not include intercourse. We ask them to focus on the physical pleasure of sexual activity and, if appropriate (when clients are not undergoing medical treatment), to refrain from intercourse during periods when conception is most likely.

We also strive to help our clients clarify the boundaries between their sexual relationship and the infertility. Many clients may need to focus their energies on rediscovering their sexual attraction for one another. One of the ways that we encourage clients to do this is to ask them to remember how they met and what initially attracted them to their partner, and to reminisce about the first stages of their relationship. For other clients, the only way to untangle the connections between infertility and their sexual relationship is temporarily or permanently to discontinue the grueling medical treatment. Ending medical treatment, even temporarily, often gives clients the freedom to do away with scheduled sex and explore expressing their sexual attraction in new ways that do not necessarily lead to intercourse.

A specific exercise we recommend calls for couples to plan dates on a weekly basis. To work effectively, the dates should be viewed as special occasions requiring planning and forethought. We ask the couple to make reservations at a favorite restaurant, shop for new clothes, or just take extra time in getting ready for the date itself. The activities themselves are less significant than the effort shown by each partner to distinguish the evening from the normal routine. When our clients can begin to focus on expressing their sexuality in their sexual relationship for the sheer pleasure of doing so, they are able to put some distance between the act of sex and the goal of pregnancy.

THE STORY OF GREG AND TRISHA

As mentioned earlier, clients who are experiencing infertility may begin to define themselves solely by the parts they play in procreation. As this definition begins to take shape, some clients disconnect from parts of their identity that are not congruent with their new perspective. For example, we have had several female clients who quit their jobs after a diagnosis of infertility so that they could focus on being a homemaker and meeting the time and energy demands of treatment. We have also worked with a large number of clients who have disconnected from their roles as an intimate partner and as a person who is comfortable expressing his or her sexual needs and desires.

The couple described in this case experienced multiple challenges in their efforts to integrate their experience with infertility into their psychosocial, sexual, and biological identities. (As we first noted in the introduction to this chapter, healthy sexuality requires the integration of all three of these elements of identity.)

Psychosocial History

Greg and Trisha entered counseling just after celebrating their fifth wedding anniversary. They described their marriage as a partnership and stated that they have tried to base their relationship on equality, communication, mutual respect, and support for one another's endeavors and life goals. Greg was an only child and Trisha was the oldest of two girls. Both were raised in single-parent families. Greg and Trisha owned and Greg managed a successful nursery and landscaping business. Trisha was a commercial real estate agent. Trisha was thirty-six and Greg was thirty-five.

This couple began trying to have a baby during the second year of their marriage. Both felt they were ready to parent and were anxious to start their family. After two years of unsuccessful attempts to get pregnant they decided to consult a specialist. The results of the fertility testing revealed that Greg had a low sperm count, and Trisha was diagnosed with "premature ovarian failure." Trisha's diagnosis basically meant that her ovaries were no longer functioning and were incapable of producing mature eggs. Greg and Trisha were told that although Greg's low sperm count would not prevent them from conceiving, Trisha's diagnosis meant that donor eggs would be necessary for a viable pregnancy.

Although Greg and Trisha were initially devastated by their prognosis and shocked that their options were so limited, we were able to help them accept that medical science could not offer them any other options for treatment. After several weeks of discussion and a consultation with a second fertility specialist, Trisha told Greg that she was unwilling to pursue the donor egg alternative.

Impact on the Relationship

Trisha based her decision not to pursue a donor program on her belief that she would not be comfortable parenting a child that was Greg's biological child but not hers. If they were unable to conceive a biological child together, she felt that they should adopt a child that was not biologically connected to either of them. Greg's response to Trisha's feelings was that he did not see the difference between Trisha's adopting his biological child and adopting a child that was not the biological child of either of them. Either way, from Greg's perspective, Trisha would not be parenting *her* biological child. Greg felt that Trisha was acting out of her grief over the loss of the biological child and believed that she needed him to be in the same position that she was.

Shortly after they were diagnosed, Greg and Trisha's differing perspectives began to be a constant source of conflict between them. Both Greg and Trisha felt that the other failed to understand their perspective. Discussions that would begin as attempts to understand one another consistently turned into full-blown arguments. The primary interaction between the two of them consisted of discussing or arguing about Trisha's decision to eliminate the donor egg program from their list of options and Greg's resentment of what he perceived as her unwillingness to consider his needs and opinions.

Prior to the infertility diagnosis, Greg and Trisha shared various interests and hobbies. Since the diagnosis and Trisha's subsequent decision, neither of them was motivated to pursue any of their mutual interests. Greg was feeling less and less motivated to attend to the details of their business, and Trisha was spending more and more time at her office. Their relationships with friends were also suffering because they didn't want to make the effort to pretend that everything was fine when in reality they were barely speaking to each other.

Clearly, Greg and Trisha's marriage was under a great deal of stress. They were not communicating, and they were distancing themselves from each other, their friends, and from pursuits that had previously been rewarding to them as individuals and as a couple. Greg and Trisha were constantly at odds with one another over this issue. When several months had gone by and Greg and Trisha were still unable to reach a compromise, they began to consider a legal separation.

Impact on Sexuality

Greg and Trisha were also experiencing a rapid loss of intimacy, and their sex life had become nonexistent. Initially their diagnosis had minimal impact on their sexual relationship. However, as the tension increased between them, their once active and mutually satisfying sexual relationship began to deteriorate. During their initial therapy session, which took place shortly after they began to consider a legal separation, Trisha described their sex life as a "battleground."

> Greg and I fight so much it doesn't surprise me that we aren't having sex anymore. Who wants to have sex with someone you're always mad at? It was really obvious to me that we were in a power struggle and that the struggle was invading our sex life. What I mean is that sex started to resemble an argument. Like Greg would want to have sex and I would say no just because he wanted to. He did the same thing to me. Sometimes it was really humiliating because one of us would initiate sex and the other person would act as though they couldn't stand the thought of being together. I just don't understand how we got to this point.

We used to share a really close and intimate relationship, but this disagreement has become the focus of our relationship. You know, there are actually times when we silently argue over the position we are having sex in. It's like a wrestling match. And whenever I was the first one to have an orgasm, Greg would get angry if I didn't immediately focus on his satisfaction. I can't tell you the number of times he accused me of being selfish—both in and out of the bedroom. It's like he can't separate me from my decision, and since my decision makes him angry, I make him angry.

Greg described the deterioration of their sexual relationship as an expected consequence of the deterioration of the trust they once had for each other.

How can we have a good relationship—sexual or otherwise—when we can't even talk to each other? She is suspicious of everything I say and do, and I don't trust her motivations either. It's like we always wonder when a thoughtful gesture or sexual experience is going to turn into a discussion about the "problem." I always find myself thinking, what is she trying to tell me or what angle is she trying to use this time? I guess I know she really isn't that devious, but we have lost all of our connections with each other, except for the infertility.

I don't see our sex life as a struggle for control, I see it as our anger spilling over into every area of our lives. I think that's because we never seem to get anywhere, and the anger just stays with us. I also think that sex is a reminder of the infertility, and the infertility is a reminder of the anger. I just don't see how things are going to get any better if we can't come to some kind of conclusion about the infertility.

Even if something suddenly changed and we could have a biological child, we are in no position to bring a child into this relationship. So, in my mind, resolving the differences comes first and a decision about the infertility comes much later. It's like we're arguing about something that we have no business doing—as if we are really ready to be parents.

This couple had reduced their relationship to the opposing sides of an argument. They were no longer able to see one another, or themselves for that matter, as individuals who are more than products of their infertility diagnosis. It is not unusual for clients to begin to view their partner and everything else in their lives through the lens of infertility. Greg and Trisha, however, engaged in this behavior to an uncommonly intense degree.

We began our work with Greg and Trisha by asking them to complete the couples inventory (included in Chapter Eleven). This exercise is intended to help our clients clarify the impact that infertility has had on their relationships. For Greg and Trisha, it was an especially important part of the therapeutic process because they had lost perspective on how influential the infertility had become in their lives.

The exercise asks clients to answer the following questions (among others):

How does the infertility affect your sexual relationship?

How does it affect your feelings about *your* role in that relationship?

How much time do you and your partner spend discussing the infertility (including treatment options, finances, reactions of others, stress points, and so on)?

What are the areas of conflict in your relationship with your partner?

In answering these questions Greg and Trisha began to realize that they were discussing infertility on a daily basis and not just with one another. They also acknowledged that their arguments about infertility had become a primary topic of discussion both between themselves and with people they were close to outside the marriage. Greg and Trisha concluded that they were spending one to two hours per day discussing the physical aspects of the infertility, the treatments, their sex life, or their perspective on the best options for them to pursue. In response to the question, What are the areas of conflict in your relationship? both Greg and Trisha listed issues surrounding sex and infertility. Their answers provided details about their disagreements regarding the best option for parenting and their feelings about the power struggle they were experiencing. Both of them talked about the resentment and mistrust that had developed between them and about their growing reluctance to have sex with each other.

Clearly, Greg and Trisha's sexual relationship had become a reflection of the dysfunction that existed in their relationship in general. Unresolved anger often manifests as a power struggle, and this was what was happening in Greg and Trisha's sexual relationship. We asked Greg and Trisha to begin having structured conversations about their anger toward each other, because for their relationship to survive, they needed to develop avenues other than their sexual relationship for the expression of anger.

As we first discussed in the case of Jason and Nancy in Chapter Three, a structured conversation is one in which each partner has fifteen minutes to explain to the other what her point of view is about anything that she feels is a problem. During each person's fifteen minutes, the other person is not supposed to do anything but listen, and ask questions if he does not understand something. Then it is the next person's turn. We tell clients that even though they may find it difficult not to interject their opinions or clarify a point, they need to remain silent, except for questions, for the full fifteen minutes. Although the initial focus for Greg and Trisha was to discuss anger, this exercise is intended ultimately to foster the development of communication skills.

We further suggested that they shift their focus to rediscovering some of their mutual interests, redeveloping intimacy in the relationship, and reconnecting with their work, family life, and friendships. We explained that these endeavors would most likely enable Greg and Trisha to regain a sense of balance in their lives and introduce other topics of conversation into their marital relationship. In therapy, we continued to focus on the primary task of reconstructing effective patterns of communication as a way to accomplish the secondary task of redeveloping a healthy sexual relationship.

In addition to continuing to encourage structured conversations, we worked on redeveloping their relationship by asking Greg and Trisha to plan dates on a weekly basis, to complete the integrity wheel (Chapter Eleven), and most important, to work through the grief about the loss of *their* potential biological children. (For more information on working through grief and loss, please see Chapter Five and the Grief and Loss sessions in Chapter Ten.)

———

In the epigraph that opens this chapter, Gloria Steinem tells us that *un*learning what we have been told about who we *should be* is essential to the development of our self-esteem. Self-esteem comes from accepting who we are, regardless of whether or not who we are is compatible with the person we have been told we should be. When clients experiencing infertility accept the infertility as one of the experiences that contribute to who they are, they foster their self-esteem. When we counsel our clients regarding difficulties with sexuality and infertility, we frequently confront the powerful influence of this society's messages about sexual expression and the roles of men and women in procreation. During our initial counseling sessions, we strive with clients to assess how these messages are influencing them and to challenge any messages they have internalized but that ultimately do not honor their true selves. This work is part of the process of unlearning.

The process of unlearning may also include challenging clients to reexamine the choices they have made about the ways in which they respond to the infertility diagnosis. Just because a coping skill has become familiar and automatic does not necessarily mean that the behavior is a healthy one. Therefore, if clients are able to unlearn the coping mechanisms that are not contributing to a healthy adjustment to this life crisis, they may be better able to develop coping skills that will facilitate their ability to have healthy sexual relationships.

Sexuality is a complicated and usually private aspect of each person's identity; it includes a lifetime of impressions, beliefs, experiences, and behaviors. Infertility is usually an unexpected intruder into our clients' already complicated sexual identity, and most clients are not prepared for the far-reaching effects of this diagnosis. To comfortably make room for this unexpected addition to their identity, our clients may need to put aside some of the ideas, beliefs, behaviors, and coping skills that existed prior to their diagnosis.

As clients begin to develop new ways of coping with an infertility diagnosis, they may also begin to reconsider their pursuit of biological parenting and to consider alternatives to biological parenting. In Chapter Seven we discuss these alternatives and the emotional factors involved in deciding to pursue them.

Considering Alternatives to Biological Parenting

We must be willing to get rid of the life we planned,
so as to have the life that is waiting for us.

—Joseph Campbell, Reflections on the Art of Living

P art of our responsibility as therapists working with clients experiencing infertility is to be aware of the available alternatives to biological parenting. Whether or not clients seek our guidance on these options, they will discuss the alternatives intermittently throughout the course of therapy. From the onset of the infertility diagnosis, it is normal for clients to begin asking What if? questions. "What if we can't have a child on our own?" "What if we decide to consider adoption?" "What if we don't have the resources to pursue treatment?" Clients ask themselves these questions whether or not they are actually at a decision-making point in their ordeal. We are therefore obligated to understand the available alternatives to biological parenting, assist clients through their decision-making process, and empower clients for effective self-advocacy. This chapter explores these issues in detail.

Before exploring the implications of each alternative to biological parenting, we must understand that an ultimate decision to pursue nonbiological parenting or child-free living does not "cure" our clients' condition of infertility. As we have previously stated, the successful outcome of these pursuits will only resolve clients' state of childlessness (even in the case of clients who choose child-free living, as they move from feeling child*less* to being child-*free*).

UNDERSTANDING THE AVAILABLE ALTERNATIVES

When traditional treatments have failed to produce a pregnancy, clients may choose to pursue advanced fertility therapies such as super-ovulation with timed intrauterine insemination (SO/IUI), gamete intrafallopian transfer (GIFT), or in vitro fertilization (IVF). Although close examination of these choices is beyond the scope of this book, we do provide information on the most commonly pursued alternatives: egg and sperm donation, surrogacy, adoption and foster care, and child-free living. The following summaries on these alternatives are provided by the American Society for Reproductive Medicine.

EGG AND SPERM DONATION

Couples with no sperm and/or eggs can undergo IVF and GIFT using donor sperm or eggs. Using a donor is a personal decision based on the couple's beliefs and the degree of their desire for a child with a biological connection to one parent. The treatment options are limited for women over 40 who have not succeeded with other therapies or for women with evidence of early menopause (premature ovarian failure). One option for older women involves the use of eggs donated by another woman. Eggs from another woman are more likely to result in pregnancy and less likely to end in miscarriage even when carried by an older woman. In the case of women who have no ovarian function due to early menopause, this treatment offers the only chance for pregnancy.

Donor sperm have been used for more than two hundred years to achieve pregnancy. Today, frozen (cryopreserved) sperm are used almost exclusively for donor insemination. Donor sperm is used only after extensive medical and genetic screening of the donor. In some cases of male infertility, fertilization may be attempted first with the male partner's sperm, and if this fails, donor sperm may be used in a second attempt. Alternatively, if several eggs are retrieved, some may be inseminated with the partner's sperm and some with donor sperm.

SURROGACY

A surrogate is a woman who agrees to become pregnant for a couple using the male partner's sperm and her own egg (traditional surrogate) or using the male partner's sperm and the female partner's egg (gestational carrier). She also agrees to give up the baby to the couple at birth. Surrogacy is a controversial option, but it can offer women over forty an opportunity to have a child who is genetically linked to the male partner. It is also an option for women who have had a hysterectomy or cannot become pregnant for medical reasons. It is critical that the surrogate be carefully screened psychologically, medically, and legally.

ADOPTION AND FOSTER CARE

Another option for having a family is adoption. Agencies have different rules regarding age and are now more receptive to older couples. There are generally no age restrictions for private adoptions. In international adoptions, some countries even prefer older parents. Foster care can offer the option to nurture a child without making a lifetime commitment, and can also help couples decide if adoption is right for them. Social Service agencies often seek couples to be foster parents.

CHILD-FREE LIVING

It is important that clients consider the option of becoming child-free if they are unable to have a biological child or if they decide to forego infertility treatment. They will need to grieve their loss and look at alternative ways to achieve new personal growth. Some people pursue a new career . . . [or] hobby, or adopt a special pet. Partners will need to discuss what is best for them.

HELPING CLIENTS THROUGH THE DECISION-MAKING PROCESS

Before clients are able to choose which alternatives to biological parenting they will pursue, they must be able to use the same decision-making skills they use under other circumstances in their lives. You can help your clients take advantage of their pragmatic problem-solving skills by using the decision-making skills exercise found in Chapter Eleven; it provides a specific format for making decisions. A sample of five questions appears here so that you can begin to see how you might direct your clients as they consider each option.

1. List all the factors (time, money, geography, schedules, emotional impact, enlisting the cooperation of others, your spouse's perspective) that you need to consider before making this decision.
2. List all the options you have to choose from. (For instance, if you are trying to decide whether or not to pursue adoption, you will include special needs, domestic, and international adoption options.)
3. What are the advantages and disadvantages of each option?
4. What are the desired outcomes of this decision?
5. What steps will you need to take to ensure those outcomes?

In addition to being able to use decision-making skills they have already demonstrated, clients must also be well-informed about their choices. The next section explores the implications of each choice so that you are equipped to prepare your clients for what each alternative involves. For a discussion that defines the options in detail and explores the practical dimensions of each choice, you can refer to Appendix C. Here we examine the decisions to stop treatment, to become child-free, to adopt, and to pursue reproductive technologies.

Deciding When to Stop Treatment

The most common reason for the discontinuation of medical treatment is the achievement of a pregnancy. Some clients, however, drift in treatment without a long-term plan. Because these clients are at risk for feeling powerless, we have developed a series of questions designed to help clients determine for themselves when enough is enough. Our exercise, when to discontinue treatment, is broken into three distinct sections that target the finances invested, the time allotted, and the events that dictate the course of medical treatment. (This exercise appears in its complete form in Chapter Eleven.)

- How much money are you willing to spend on infertility treatment?

  Are you willing to spend your savings?

  Are you willing to incur debt?

  Are you willing to jeopardize your medical insurability?

• What will it take for you to know, regardless of new technologies, that you are finished with all attempts to conceive through medical intervention?

You must achieve a pregnancy and carry to full term.

Your physician tells you there is nothing more that can be done.

Your partner tells you that the relationship is at risk.

You have used all of your financial resources.

You have (or your partner has) experienced menopause.

You decide to consider the alternatives to biological parenting.

You realize that your life has become consumed by infertility and that you want more than this for yourself and your partner.

If you are working with partners in a relationship, both clients should be given these questions as homework for completion before the next scheduled session. Ask each partner to complete their own questionnaire and then discuss their responses with one another when they are done. You can use the results of the exercise, and any decisions the clients have reached, to launch the next therapy hour. If you are working with just one partner, you might consider using the exercise in session so that your client has an opportunity to process the questions with you. You can then discuss ways in which your client can convey his answers to his partner outside the therapeutic setting.

The answers to the questions are not as important as your clients' ability to make a decision and commit to that decision. Your support, combined with your clients' ability to follow through with the plan they have designed for themselves, will demonstrate the power in taking responsibility for their own well-being. Without a long-term plan, clients drifting in treatment can end up pursuing treatment obsessively.

Some clients reach a point in their infertility treatment where they become preoccupied with feelings of being different, inferior, and isolated. These clients are unable to think of anything but the desire to have a baby so that they can be included in the broader culture's experience of family life. This preoccupation constitutes a serious cause for concern because it suggests that these clients are overlooking all other areas of their lives. As these clients' overall functioning diminishes, they withdraw psychologically and emotionally from everything except the quest to become pregnant. They believe that this quest is the only thing that gives their life meaning.

When clients' reproductive systems fail to respond to the myriad treatments they have endured, the preoccupation with their feelings of being different, inferior, and isolated can evolve into an obsession with conquering infertility. This obsession manifests as a crusade to triumph over the odds of success of the latest available reproductive technology. Clients with an extreme form of this obsession, determined to prove that *they* will be the miracle patient, engage in an aggressive, competitive battle with their physicians.

Obsession is a persistent idea, desire, or emotion that cannot be resolved by reasoning. To obsess is to haunt or trouble in mind to an abnormal degree. We believe that obsessions become the eyes with which clients see the world. The obsession with conquering infertility can cause clients to feel as though every woman on the street is pregnant and every couple has children, except them.

Obsessed clients lose their normal reasoning abilities and feel compelled to submit to countless surgical procedures, general anaesthesia, and daily injections over the course of several years. During one counseling session, a client lifted her baggy shorts to reveal her black-and-blue thighs. They were so severely bruised from her daily Pergonal injections that it was hard for us to look at them. The client said, "I'm so glad summer is finally here and I can wear these loose-fitting shorts. It's impossible to find baggy pants that will keep me warm in the winter. And there are no pants, dresses, or skirts that don't put pressure on the bruising." Although this particular client expressed her embarrassment over the appearance of her body, she willingly revealed her thighs as a heroic soldier might show a battle scar or war wound. This client seemed to view her physical distortions as evidence of her participation in the infertility treatment battle.

Another client lifted her shirt without warning to reveal extensive abdominal scarring. If we had not known that the scars were a result of surgical procedures that attempted to correct the infertility, we might have assumed that the scars had been inflicted in a brutal attack or incurred through a serious accident. This client's gesture of raising her shirt, without inhibition, was suggestive of a pregnant woman proudly revealing her swollen belly. It was as if this client, in her subconscious struggle to find meaning in her disfigurement, identified the consequence of her *infertility* with the consequence of a pregnant woman's *fertility*, as if to say, "Look what I have. I deserve attention and have worth, too."

We are frequently moved by what some clients are compelled to go through, all in the name of procreation. We believe that clients' obsessive pursuit of medical treatment is an attempt to overcompensate for their feelings of powerlessness. The course of medical treatment appears to be a path on which clients can exercise choice, but the outcome of treatment is still a factor over which clients have little control.

Some members of Alcoholics Anonymous, the original twelve-step program, define the "insanity" mentioned in step two as repeating the same behavior over and over again and expecting a different result. By using this definition we do not mean to say that some clients are insane, but that their behaviors are. The choice to pursue medical intervention with blinding vehemence, after years of no success, is insane. Many clients readily admit, "I know I'm crazy, but I don't care." The frenzy with which obsessed clients continue to pursue treatment, exacerbated by the constant advances in medical technology, can perpetuate serious denial of these clients' predicament.

The fertility treatment industry unwittingly nurtures these clients' obsession with biological parenting. The industry is challenged and motivated to find a solution to clients' fertility problems. It is therefore understandable that a physician's drive to help, combined with a client's obsession, can prohibit the infertility specialist from seeing the client's *emotional* struggle with infertility. In these cases, we can help clients to step back, and we can help them to determine when enough is enough. As we suggested earlier, one way you can do this by using the when to discontinue treatment exercise. The third section of the exercise follows. You can use this section to help your clients see what it is they might be sacrificing as they obsessively pursue infertility treatment:

• How long are you willing to undergo treatment?

For how many months or years will you endure physical discomfort?

For how many months or years will you forfeit your privacy?

For how many months or years will you compromise your sexual freedom?

For how many months or years will you compromise your psychological and emotional well-being?

Without the opportunity to look at the emotional, financial, and psychological costs of treatment, clients will inevitably fall into a pattern of behaviors that are incongruent with reality. Therapeutic intervention is imperative in these cases, and must focus on regaining perspective and establishing manageable limits. Otherwise, clients in obsessive pursuit of medical treatment invest everything (emotionally, financially, and psychologically) in a prospective pregnancy and are subsequently unable to see other options that are available to them.

Deciding to Become Child-Free

Many clients hear the term *child-free* and assume that it must be the politically correct or euphemistic way of referring to people who are *childless*. Underlying this assumption is the belief that no one would ever *choose* not to have children. Thus, for most clients, becoming child-free is a process by which they evolve from seeing themselves as childless to embracing a child-free lifestyle. Clients who describe themselves as child-free have grieved for the loss of the imagined child, examined the short-and long-term implications of a life without traditional parenting, and affirmed the life they can go on to lead. (For the purposes of this discussion, we use two definitions of parenting. Traditional parenting is defined as permanently providing nurturing and modeling for children who live in the home, and assuming financial, legal, and moral responsibility for those children. Traditional parenting includes biological and adoptive parenting. We define nontraditional parenting as temporarily fulfilling any or all of the responsibilities fulfilled by traditional parents. Nontraditional parenting includes godparenting, foster parenting, and other capacities in which adults may act as significant role models in the life of a child.)

We must emphasize that choosing to be child-free is not the same as rejecting children. Rather, child-free living is a positive, life-affirming choice. Clients are child-free voluntarily, whereas by remaining childless clients define themselves by what they do not have and obviously want.

Because most clients do not grow up hearing "child-free living" uttered as an option, most clients assume that they will become parents and have never considered the possibility of not becoming parents. This is one reason why an infertility diagnosis can be such a blow to clients' expectations about their life. Clients can become motivated to conquer the *condition,* and they lose the ability to ask themselves if the pursuit of a child is really what they want and in their best interest. Some clients have remarked that it is as if they feverishly pursue a pregnancy because they know they cannot achieve one.

When clients do begin to consider child-free living, they often grapple with the expectations of others in their life. Clients know that they might be viewed as selfish and unable to carry out what is considered the most important task of adulthood, because they have had these same thoughts about themselves and others they know who are child-free. We now explore how clients can deal with cultural expectations, redefine parenting, and consider the realistic implications of child-free living.

FACING CULTURAL EXPECTATIONS.   Our clients tell us that it is very challenging to be child-free in a child-focused society. They have the most difficulty dealing with two widely held tenets: (1) raising children is the primary task of adulthood, and (2) the most significant, tangible contribution to the world is evidenced through child bearing and rearing.

Our child-free clients point out that our culture's definition of family necessarily includes children. These clients are frustrated because the union they create with their partner is not acknowledged as a family unit. Child-free couples want to be understood as well-adjusted, complete families who are fulfilling *other* primary tasks of adulthood.

When faced with the news of the success of their peers' children, child-free clients can feel directly confronted by cultural expectations because they will bear no child who might find an important cure or contribute to world peace. We have created an exercise called considering child-free living that includes an exploration of other tangible contributions to the human race. A part of this exercise is included here so that you can consider how you might begin to reframe this predicament for your clients. (The complete exercise appears in Chapter Eleven.)

1. Were you hoping to contribute something tangible to the world?
   a. How else can you contribute to the world?
   b. Have you considered any of the following?
      • Writing a book, newsletter, or article for publication
      • Setting up a trust fund for a friend or relative's child

- Creating or contributing to a scholarship fund at a university or college
- Helping to fund a public human service agency
- Participating in a research project sponsored by a local college
- Sponsoring a child overseas with small monthly contributions
- Volunteering for a nonprofit organization

REDEFINING PARENTING.   Being child-free does not mean that clients cannot be actively involved with children or even participate in a nontraditional parenting role (as defined earlier). The ability of our child-free clients to redefine parenting has allowed them to become *more* involved with children, where they once avoided this type of contact. Whereas engaging in infertility treatment emphasized clients' childlessness, embracing child-free living allows these same clients to let go of their jealousy and resentment. Because they have embraced their own lives, they become able to embrace the milestones and celebrations of others. Clients are ultimately able to define the meaning of their own role in the lives of the children they care about. (For a more comprehensive discussion of this process, see the Alternatives to Biological Parenting session in Chapter Ten.)

Some of our clients have chosen to play active roles in the lives of their nieces, nephews, and godchildren, and the children of friends. Others have become involved in Big Brother and Big Sister programs, scouting programs, Little League coaching, and religious youth groups. These clients report that they are able to include some of these children on special outings and vacations. Some clients choose to provide temporary care to foster children or emergency shelter for runaways and other troubled youths. By redefining parenting, child-free clients are able to deflect the criticism that they are selfish. These clients, who demonstrate the primary characteristics of parenting, essentially become nontraditional parents who are often praised for their devotion to others' children.

Child-free clients who are able to recreate the meaning of the parenting role seem comfortable with their fit into the broader culture. Where they once felt that not being traditional eliminated them from the broader culture, their role as active, nurturing role models for the children in their lives fulfills a great need. In addition to meeting the needs of specific children, child-free clients are able to pursue other interests with the passion and vigor they experienced prior to their infertility diagnosis. Unlike clients who expect children to give meaning to their lives and relationship, these child-free clients have developed their identities separate from the children who rely on them to fulfill a certain role.

CONSIDERING REALISTIC IMPLICATIONS.   Clients who choose a child-free lifestyle report that they enjoy several advantages over their friends who are traditional parents. They report that they have the time and energy to pursue lifelong ambitions such as world travel and artistic endeavors. In addition, child-free living may lead to greater satisfaction in marriages. A recent study by the American Sociological Association, reported on *Good Morning America,* showed that marital satisfaction decreases with the addition of each child to the family. This study and others like it point to the difficulty in maintaining healthy, growing marriages when the demands of children are immediate, constant, and long term. With children in the home, partners often may delay or neglect meeting each other's needs or those of the marriage. Child-free couples have the freedom to respond to one another on a consistent basis and to pursue individual needs without sacrificing marital satisfaction.

Child-free clients also note the financial freedom they experience. They have fewer expenses and have the freedom to earn less money than their peers who are traditional parents. These clients also have the flexibility to take more risks in their employment positions, including relocating, making career changes, pursuing advanced degrees, and reducing their hours. These clients know they are not obligated to maintain certain positions because they have dependents who rely on them to provide basic needs.

At various points in their lives, clients who choose to embrace a child-free life may experience a resurgence of the sadness about the loss of their biological child. We explore the resurgence of grief in Chapter Eight. We mention the inevitability of resurfacing grief now to remind you that child-free living does not *resolve* the clients' infertility experience. Rather, child-free living is an alternative to biological parenting that can also be an alternative to traditional parenting.

Deciding to Adopt

Clients who are experiencing infertility may also decide to pursue parenting through adoption; they have three basic types of adoption to choose from: domestic, international, and special needs. Many variations exist within each type of adoption, and sometimes one adoption can incorporate aspects of more than one type. Please refer to Appendix C for a discussion that defines each type of adoption and examines the factors that are common and unique to each type of adoption. Here we discuss the implications of parenting children who are adopted.

IMPLICATIONS OF PARENTING CHILDREN ADOPTED DOMESTICALLY.   Clients who are considering domestic special needs or transracial or transcultural adoption will need to face the same issues that are discussed in the special needs section of this chapter. Aside from the parenting issues of special needs and transracial and transcultural adoptions, domestic adoptions often involve parenting issues related to ongoing openness between adoptive and birth parents.

Potential adoptive parents often make decisions about contact with birth parents before they fully understand the implications of that contact. Some potential adoptive parents are quite comfortable with openness and do not hesitate to engage in an open relationship with potential birth parents. Others are uncomfortable with openness but hesitate to refuse contact with birth parents. These clients often feel that if they refuse contact the birth parents may reject them as potential parents for their child. Other adoptive parents realize that openness is an inherent part of the initial stages of some types of adoption, such as a private adoption facilitated through an advertisement, but do not realize that birth parents may desire the same levels of contact after a child is placed that they had during the pregnancy.

Adoptive parents will face lifelong consequences of their initial decisions about the level of openness in any adoption they pursue. In the best-case scenario, adoptive and birth parents will reach an understanding with which they are both comfortable. In the worst case, adoptive parents will make commitments to openness that they later decide they cannot keep. For adoptive parents who have a high degree of openness with birth parents, a primary concern will be to integrate the birth parents into their relationship with their adopted child.

In open relationships, adoptive parents will need to explain to the child both the presence of the birth parents and the child's relationship to the birth parents. This explanation can be complicated and confusing, but it can be done. The key for adoptive parents is to give their child age-appropriate information and to answer their child's questions in an honest and clear way. There can be many benefits to this type of relationship when birth parents are respectful of the child's needs and all parties act in the best interest of the child. (If the birth parents are unable or unwilling to act in the child's best interest, adoptive parents must make whatever decisions they feel are appropriate.) One of the benefits of an open relationship is the elimination of the mystery surrounding the birth parents, for both the child and the adoptive parents. When a positive relationship exists between the adoptive and birth parents, the child can incorporate the adoptive parents' positive attitudes about the child's genetic identity into his self-concept.

In adoptive relationships in which commitments to birth parents are broken because of the adoptive parents' discomfort with openness, the adoptive parents are faced with explaining those broken commitments to the child. If the adoptive parents keep their decisions secret and the child eventually discovers the truth, the child will experience a break in trust with her adoptive parents. The bottom line for adoptive parents, then, is to consider not only what they are comfortable with but also how they will explain their decisions to their child. There are many resources available to adoptive parents on the issue of openness; Adoptive Families of America can provide a list of those resources. (See Appendix B for information on this organization.)

IMPLICATIONS OF PARENTING CHILDREN ADOPTED INTERNATIONALLY.
We recommend that our clients educate themselves about the country from which they are adopting. We ask that clients read political, economic, and cultural accounts of the country's history and that they consider studying the language, culinary art, and fine art of their prospective child's country of origin. Education facilitates understanding and respect for the entire collage of influences that contribute to their child's development. With the newly acquired knowledge, clients are in a position to support their children as the unique individuals they are.

Many foreign-born children available for adoption are members of a minority race; over one year of age; have medical, emotional, or psychological problems; or have experienced developmental delays and are therefore classified as children with special needs. We empha-size the special needs of foreign-born children because many clients, adoption professionals, and mental health practitioners believe that children adopted internationally do not necessarily present special needs. On the contrary, foreign-born children will *always* present spe-cial needs to their adoptive parents by virtue of the circumstances that allow international adoptions to occur at all. These children are in need of homes due to extreme poverty, war, and the sending country's inability to meet the children's needs in time to ensure that they will survive. Furthermore, clients who pursue parenting through interna-tional adoption need to consider that transracial and transcultural placements challenge adoptive parents to support their child's unique origins on an *ongoing basis.*

Prospective adoptive parents must consider how they will provide positive role models in order to support their child's developing iden-tity. Clients also need to examine their views of the sending country in order to address any negative judgments they may hold as facts; they must develop understanding and compassion for a country that looks to other countries for assistance in crisis. This view epitomizes the ultimate commitment parents can make to their child's well-being.

IMPLICATIONS OF PARENTING CHILDREN WITH SPECIAL NEEDS. One of the key components of the home study (a written evaluation of the potential parents' suitability for adoptive parenting) is educating the client. We provide comprehensive information about the specific is-sues that parents need to consider when adopting a child with special needs. For both domestic and international adoptions, we ask clients to complete an adoption worksheet (Chapter Eleven). This worksheet lists numerous conditions that may be present in the child or in the birth parent's medical and social history. The form asks clients to con-sider whether they are able to accept a child who has specific issues in his background that may influence the child's physical, emotional, or psychological development. Examples of children with special needs include the following:

• A child who is over the age of two. Clients must consider their ability to parent a child whose habits, preferences, and ideas are already forming or formed. They must ask themselves if they are able to substitute guidance in place of influence over their devel-oping child.

- A child who has been abused, neglected, or both. Clients must consider what they expect of their child. Children who have been abused or neglected may act out or be unable to feel or express love for their adoptive parents. Clients must therefore ask themselves whether they hope to have their love returned by their children or whether they can be satisfied simply by providing support to their child.

- A child who has medical problems. Clients must consider the short- and long-term implications of nutritional delays, congenital defects, and sustained injuries. They must ask themselves whether they expect to correct problems or are willing to accept uncorrectable conditions and help their child maximize her greatest potential, despite physical limitations.

Some special needs adoptions also involve transcultural and transracial placements. In these cases, we ask that prospective parents examine their own prejudices as well as the attitudes that are pervasive in their extended families and their professional and social circles. Many clients will state that they could parent *any* child, but the interview process reveals that their lifestyle does not demonstrate support of *every* child. We ask clients to consider their friends, the neighborhood they live in, and whom they see in their community. For instance, clients who live in culturally and racially diverse communities are often better prepared to parent a child with a different ethnicity from their own. Clients who live in relatively homogeneous communities will be more challenged to explain to their child the absence of others like him.

All parents adopting children from different races and cultures or children with medical challenges need to provide positive role models for their children. Ideally, these models should be integrated into the family as opposed to conspicuously placed as same-race or same-condition models in their child's life just to demonstrate support. Adoptive parents are responsible for demonstrating that their family composition, although unique, exists elsewhere and that it is only one of all the possible family compositions. Parents can demonstrate their family's normalcy through their membership and attendance in community support groups. Ideally, children with special needs will see themselves *reflected* in the broader community and sense that they *belong* in the broader community.

Clients who adopt a child with special needs must also expect to have those special needs trigger specific memories of their infertility experience at various points in their child's development. One example might be a daughter who at six years of age was placed with her adoptive parents as a result of being sexually abused. It is common for children with a history of sexual abuse to act at the onset of adolescence in ways that are considered promiscuous. If, at fifteen years of age, the daughter announces that she is pregnant and intends to have an abortion, her adoptive parents may reexperience their own grief about the biological child they could never have. In order to parent effectively and guide their daughter in her own life-altering event, adoptive parents must first confront their own grief issues. We discuss the management of resurfacing grief at length in Chapter Eight.

Deciding to Pursue Reproductive Technologies

Because some procedures are not medically appropriate for all clients, the decision to pursue a particular treatment is often determined by the results of specific tests. Each procedure also carries various implications for clients who decide to pursue one of these options. The following sections examine the emotional dimensions of selecting a donor alternative and the implications of parenting a child who is conceived through one of these procedures.

SELECTING A DONOR ALTERNATIVE.   When clients decide to pursue medical alternatives to biological parenting, they must often consider an overwhelming amount of information. Clients must sift through medical information, variances in state laws, and information about individual donor programs. At the same time, clients must comprehend the technical nature of much of this information. For a discussion of the practical considerations for selecting a donor alternative, please refer to Appendix C. The following discussion explores the emotional factors to consider.

CONSIDERING EMOTIONAL FACTORS.   The most common emotional issues that couples face during the selection of a donor alternative are related to the loss of the potential biological child of one or both partners, and the relationships among the parenting couple, the child, and the donor or surrogate.

Loss of the Potential Biological Child of One or Both Partners.   As we discussed in Chapter Five, the loss of the potential biological child can be extremely difficult for clients to work through and accept. When clients pursue donor programs such as embryo adoption, both partners may experience grief about the loss of the potential biological child. Donor alternatives that use either donor sperm or donor eggs will result in only one partner experiencing the loss of a genetic connection to the couple's child. Both partners, however, will experience the loss of a jointly conceived biological child.

Each of these client losses is unique but can nonetheless be addressed through our model of grief therapy. (Refer to Chapter Five for additional information about using our model with couples experiencing infertility.) The therapist should clarify the distinctions between each partner's losses and the couple's joint losses, and deal with them as separate issues. For clients to accept the loss of the potential biological child, they must first learn to cope with their own grief and the grief of their partner. When grief work is successful, clients are able to integrate the loss of the potential biological child into their present, individual identities, as well as into their identity as a couple. However, clients should understand that grief and integration are lifelong issues that will be shaped by their future circumstances and stages of life.

Relationships Between the Parenting Couple, the Child, and the Donor or Surrogate.   Clients are often confused about what type of relationship they want to have with the donor or surrogate; clients wonder whether the relationship should be ongoing, when and if the child should be included in the relationship, and how to explain the relationship to the child. Sometimes one or more of these decisions are predetermined because the donor program is anonymous. However, not all donors remain anonymous, and many clients must deal with these relationship issues. In addition, clients must begin to make these decisions before they fully understand the implications for themselves and their child. A lack of understanding of the long-term implications of these relationships may foster further confusion and anxiety.

We recommend that clients begin the decision-making process by educating themselves about the advantages and disadvantages of these relationships. We encourage clients to educate themselves through reading and conversations with other parents who have been through similar situations. We then suggest that clients limit their commitments for contact with the donor or surrogate to a degree with which they are comfortable and to a designated time frame that seems manageable to them. For clients who are unsure about their ability to follow through on commitments to ongoing contact, we further recommend that they select a program that leaves future contact up to their discretion.

After clients develop an initial relationship with their donor or surrogate and begin to parent, they are better able to evaluate the implications of these relationships and to make realistic decisions about them. The parenting couple needs to make decisions about ongoing relationships with the donor or surrogate within the context of their evolving needs and those of their child. For instance, not all children will want contact with the surrogate parents. On the other hand, some surrogates become an extraordinarily positive influence in the lives of the children to whom they helped give life. Clients may therefore wish to broaden their relationship with the donor or to limit it according to their beliefs about what is in the best interest of the child. In any event, clients will be best served by a program that anticipates that their clients' needs may change over time and that has the flexibility to adjust to those changing needs.

We always recommend that clients be honest with their child about the circumstances of their conception and any contact that they have had with the donor or surrogate. The information that parents share with their child should be age appropriate and can be incorporated into other discussions about reproduction, sexuality, and the various ways in which children come into families. As children grasp these concepts and develop emotional maturity, we recommend that parents offer additional information to them. Children cope most effectively with information that they are given over time, in age-appropriate doses; they cope less effectively with information that they are given in a formal, "sit down, we have something to tell you" conversation (especially if that information has been kept from children for a long period of time).

When clients are considering *not* telling their child about the circumstances of her conception, they must be cautioned about the possibility that the child may find out on her own. Because family members, neighbors, coworkers, and friends of the couple often know about their plans to adopt or use a donor, it is quite likely that the information could inadvertently get back to the child through one of these sources. In addition, one of our colleagues who practices family law tells us that it is not unheard of for the circumstances of a child's conception to become an issue in divorce cases. In court, he has repeatedly seen evidence presented that the biological parent of a child conceived with the assistance of a donor has used the other parent's lack of biological connection to the child to alienate the child from the nonbiological parent. In light of the fact that over 50 percent of all marriages in the United States end in divorce, it is not presumptuous to assume that some of our clients may be involved in a similar scenario.

We have also worked with a number of adult adoptees who have come across their original adoption paperwork when going through a deceased parent's files and papers, and we have worked with teenagers who have "come across" adoption paperwork in their parents' files and thus discovered their adoptive status. Needless to say, when children (be they preteens, teenagers, or adults) inadvertently discover a secret of this magnitude, it can cause a severe breach of trust between them and their adoptive parents.

The emotional implications of a challenge to the client's rights to parent will inevitably be tied to the client's original reproductive losses. Previous losses commonly resurface with the occurrence of another loss. Although a challenge by a surrogate to the termination of her parental rights may not result in legal alterations to the original contract, clients will still experience a grief reaction to the potential loss of the fulfillment of their dreams about parenting this child. Their grief reaction will be compounded by their attachment to the child, developed throughout the pregnancy (regardless of whether or not the female partner in the relationship actually carried the pregnancy); their physical contact with the child (including primary care of the child, holding and physically expressing their feelings for the child, and their presence in the delivery room); and their attachment to and trust of the surrogate (which clients will most likely feel has been violated).

You can help your clients cope with the stressors in these situations. You can assist your clients by encouraging them to advocate on their own behalf and on behalf of their child's best interests. Clients may want to seek the support of other parents who have experienced similar situations, facilitate civil mediation between them and the surrogate, or work through their fears about continuing to develop bonds with the child when they are faced with the possibility of losing their legal rights to parent. (This is especially challenging when clients have physical custody of the child but are unsure of their continued ability to retain that custody.)

Whatever the outcome of the legal dispute, clients will need to work through the implications of having gone through it. Clients will need either to accept the loss of the child if the court awards custody to the surrogate, learn to work with a surrogate who has been granted visitation rights to a child, or work through any negative feelings toward the surrogate (to minimize the impact of these feelings on their relationship with the child) if the court terminates the legal rights of the surrogate parent and awards custody to your clients.

As you can see, the introduction of a donor into the process of infertility treatment further complicates the process of reproduction for clients who are experiencing infertility. Before deciding to become parents through any donor alternative, clients need to consider the emotional implications we have discussed. As potential parents explore their alternatives to biological parenting, we best serve our clients if we have a basic understanding of the available reproductive technologies and the emotional factors that are most likely to affect the client's decision to pursue a donor alternative.

EMPOWERING CLIENTS FOR EFFECTIVE SELF-ADVOCACY

We began this chapter by suggesting that clients have usually begun to educate themselves about alternatives to biological parenting prior to their initial session with us. Our reason for providing you with the information your clients probably already have is to help you effectively guide and support your clients during their search for the appropriate alternative to biological parenting. Although it is necessary that you have relevant information and are able to explore the emotional dimensions of each alternative with your clients (discussed in this chapter), we suggest that you refrain from providing your clients with facts in areas where they have gaps in their information. In order to foster your clients' ability to be effective self-advocates, we recommend that you be able to broker information and promote assertiveness so that your clients can themselves acquire information that might be difficult to obtain.

Brokering Information

As we mentioned in Chapter Two, you must be able to provide relevant resources to your clients. If you can successfully refer your clients to other professionals and appropriate lay people who meet clients' complex and diverse needs throughout the infertility experience, your clients will come to trust that you are knowledgeable and genuinely interested in their well-being. Furthermore, your clients' capacity to have their needs met by numerous individuals will demonstrate that they need not rely on any one source (including you) to help them navigate the experience of infertility. You can, in effect, become your clients' touchstone for all the services they receive, and are in a position to help them assess the paths they want to explore.

Your clients inevitably become empowered when they can take what you give them and ascertain whether or not it is acceptable to them. One way for you to promote this empowerment is to provide them with more than one source for each request—for example, the names of three attorneys for an investigation of the legal implications of surrogate parenting. This way your clients can ultimately choose for themselves which resource is the best match for them. In Appendix B, we provide a list of resources that can help your clients begin the process of acquiring information they want and do not have.

Once clients choose an alternative, they need to contact the program or agency they are considering and ask to speak with other clients who have used the program's services and agreed to serve as references. Clients should also check the program's record with the Better Business Bureau, the attorney general's office, and local support groups in the state or city in which the program operates. Clients should note the program representatives' responses to their questions, whether or not any commitments for return calls and program information were responded to in a timely manner, and their overall impression of the program's customer service. From these notes, clients should be able to form a relatively sound judgment about the quality of the agency's or program's relationship with its clients.

Promoting Assertiveness

Sometimes clients have difficulty acquiring information even if the sources they have been given are reliable and appropriate. As we have mentioned throughout this book, some clients who experience infertility feel powerless and unable to influence their experience. We have worked with numerous clients who are afraid to ask physicians specific questions regarding their diagnosis, treatment, and prognosis. Some clients state that they do not wish to "bother" their doctors; others forget to ask questions during their visits and assume it is inappropriate to phone their physicians outside of their allotted times. We had one client who was convinced that if she asked too many questions, her physician would not be as committed to helping her achieve a pregnancy.

We help our clients develop assertiveness by asking them to look at other areas in their lives in which they would not think twice about getting the information they want or need. One client, for example, commented that she would never be afraid to "bother" her car mechanic for information, because she knew that both her safety and her money might be at risk if she did not ask the appropriate questions, yet she was unable to ask her doctor about the side effects she might experience while taking a new fertility drug.

You should encourage your clients to approach selecting a program as consumers who need to be educated about their options, rather than as potential clients whose prospects for parenting are in the hands of agency or program staff. When clients view themselves as consumers, they are more likely to recognize that they are entitled to answers to their questions and information about the program they are considering. For instance, if clients perceive that the facilitators of a program are not receptive to answering questions or require the client to be conciliatory in order to be accepted into the program, we advocate that the clients should eliminate that program from consideration. We take this stand because we believe that the staff of donor programs should not foster client disempowerment and vulnerability. You may need to demonstrate and provide training in the use of skills that will enable clients to be assertive during the process of selecting an alternative to biological parenting. (Please refer to the Self-Advocacy session in Chapter Ten for more information.)

In this chapter, we explored options for clients who have been diagnosed with fertility problems and are considering alternatives to biological parenting. Clients may decide to pursue parenting with the assistance of reproductive technologies, to adopt, or to be child-free. As we have seen, each of the alternatives has emotional implications for our clients. Therefore, before deciding which alternatives they will pursue, our clients should fully explore the emotional aspects of each choice. (Clients also should explore the practical implications of each option, and we have included this discussion in Appendix C.)

In addition to Appendix C and the information provided in this chapter, we have also included a list of resources (Appendix B). These resources provide both you and your clients with educational materials, support, newsletters, and referral services that supplement the information in this chapter.

CHAPTER EIGHT

Coping with Recurring Grief and Doubt

You cannot step twice into the same river; for other and ever other rivers flow on.

—*Heracleitus*

In Chapter One, we expressed our view that it is impossible to resolve grief. An individual's infertility experience can lay dormant as a subconscious memory. Any new stressor can cause the memories, and all the accompanying reactions to the experience of infertility (such as anger, sadness, and confusion), to bring the old grief and doubt up into consciousness. This grief and doubt usually resurfaces in conjunction with life events or comments from others; the event or comment may not appear on the surface to be directly linked to the client's experience with infertility, but on a deeper level, it may trigger a reexamination of previous life decisions, or emotions similar to those associated with the infertility experience. And although the feelings and thoughts are similar to those experienced in the initial ordeal, there are two important distinctions between initial grief and resurfacing grief. First, recurring grief is *experienced differently* than is initial grief; second, when grief and doubt resurface, clients usually *manage the experience differently* than they did the first time.

Although recurring grief is overwhelming and difficult, clients experience it differently than they do initial grief. With initial grief, clients may wonder what is happening to them and question whether they will be able to get through the experience. When grief and doubt resurface, clients have the benefit of having already experienced the host of emotions and thoughts that accompany grief. Though no more welcome in their lives than the first time, the grief is usually an understood experience, and clients have the benefit of knowing that they have survived it once and will do so again.

This understanding can allow clients to let go and experience resurfacing grief, whereas during the initial episode clients were likely to have resisted the experience of grief. Clients also are usually able to manage their grief differently in subsequent episodes because they have (ideally) developed a repertoire of helpful coping mechanisms. They are not as likely to struggle with trying to understand what works for them and what does not. In addition to your clients' increased self-awareness developed from the initial grief, you will have the advantage of being able to draw on the former experience when your clients may not have the clarity to do so. You might, for example, ask such questions as, "Were there any rituals that you found helpful that you could reconstruct?" or "What support systems did you have in place last time?" You can bring all of your clients' coping mechanisms into play to help clients navigate resurfacing grief and doubt, regardless of what event provokes the experience.

This chapter examines six categories of potential stressors that may cause clients to experience resurfacing grief and doubt: (1) anticipated life events, (2) unanticipated life events, (3) other people's lack of awareness, (4) changes in sexual functioning, (5) parenting stages, and (6) the fertility of others. We also provide strategies for treating your clients when they experience resurfacing grief and doubt related to the infertility ordeal.

ANTICIPATED LIFE EVENTS

Expected life events may trigger the memory of the infertility experience. Regardless of whether clients have time to plan for the event or not, they are usually surprised by the resurgence of grief and doubt over the infertility experience. Nonetheless, you can prepare clients for the likelihood of the resurgence, so they are at least able to recognize what is happening when it occurs. Some of the anticipated life events that can cause grief to resurface include anniversaries of previous losses, the death of a loved one, menopause, and retirement.

Anniversaries of Previous Losses

Anniversaries of losses that clients experienced as a result of their infertility diagnosis—a stillbirth, a miscarriage, a final treatment procedure—can trigger grief. Anniversaries of losses not associated with the infertility (such as the anniversary of a parent's, friend's, or spouse's death) can remind clients of other losses they have suffered, including those associated with the infertility.

You can prepare your clients for these reactions and discuss in advance what they can do to cope with their feelings of sadness, loss, or anger. We suggest that clients mark anniversaries with rituals that have meaning for them. Clients may choose to visit a grave site or spend time alone reflecting on the relationship or the events surrounding the loss. It is the acknowledgment of the loss and acceptance of the accompanying emotions and not *how* they acknowledge the loss that are essential to continued growth and healing.

Death of a Loved One

Whether or not clients have had time to prepare for the death of their loved one, they are likely to be caught off guard by the reemergence of their memories of the infertility experience. The case that follows illustrates the confusion some clients experience when the memory of the infertility ordeal resurfaces.

Andrea and Casey reinitiated therapy after Andrea's mother died. The couple had adopted a sibling set of two: a two-year-old girl and a three-year-old boy from Russia. They pursued adoption after five years of infertility treatment and two years of evaluating all the alternatives to biological parenting. Andrea and Casey had been parenting their children for two years when Andrea's mother died after a long battle with cancer.

ANDREA: My mom's death has been real hard on me. I miss her and the kids miss her. I am so sad and down most of the time. I thought I was prepared; she had been sick for so long. The thing that concerns me the most is that I keep thinking about all the infertility treatments. I do not know what that has to do with my mother's death. I thought that was all over anyway. We could not have asked for two better kids than the ones we have. I need some help getting through this.

CASEY: And I do not know how to help because I keep thinking about everything we went through trying to get pregnant, too. We thought we had better come in and find out if it is normal to have all these unrelated memories come back to us while we are trying to get used to Andrea's mom being gone.

THERAPIST: It is interesting that you both express that the memories of the infertility experience seem unrelated to the death of the kids' grandma. Why do you think you might be having these memories at this time?

CASEY: Well, I do not really know. I do know that the sadness about both things feels pretty much the same.

ANDREA: I have that sense, too. That somehow the infertility experience and my mother's death are connected, but I do not know how they are connected.

THERAPIST: Sometimes sadness over losses experienced long ago comes up when new loss is experienced. So, what did you lose with infertility?

ANDREA: Our biological child.

THERAPIST: And what did you lose with the death of Andrea's mother?

ANDREA: My mom and a grandparent to our children.

THERAPIST: With each experience, you lost something very special to you.

CASEY: That is interesting. I can see that the infertility was really about a death, too. It brought the death of a dream.

THERAPIST: Yes. And did any dreams die with the death of your mother-in-law?

CASEY: Well, yes. The dream of an ongoing relationship with her and the kids.

ANDREA: That is true. And now I am thinking that I feel sad because my mom never got to have *biological* grandchildren. All this time *we* have been OK with that, but I never asked my mom if *she* was OK with that. Not only have I lost the opportunity to ask her, but I will never know the answer. Now I feel just as inadequate as a daughter as I felt as a woman when I could not get pregnant.

Although the loss of Andrea's mother was an anticipated loss for this couple, they did not expect to feel renewed sadness about their infertility experience. Nor did they know that an old loss could be experienced in new ways, as with Andrea's discoveries that her infertility might have been experienced as a loss by her mother and that her feelings of inadequacy could expand into new arenas. Most clients are able to cope with the reemergence of their grief over the infertility once they understand its relevance to the new loss. We encouraged Andrea to begin a journal (guidelines provided in Chapter Eleven) so that she could express her grief over both losses, and work through her feelings of inadequacy and regret.

Menopause

The onset of menopause can trigger the reemergence of feelings associated with your clients' original reproductive losses. Because menopause marks the end of the childbearing years, couples who were unable to conceive through reproductive technologies must face the end of the chances of a "miracle" pregnancy and of having biological children. The miracle pregnancy is the last hope for many clients who have experienced infertility, have never been given a definitive answer about the cause of the infertility, have ended treatment, and are still hoping that without intervention they may beat the odds and get pregnant on their own. Although most clients do not rely on this possibility, many clients tell us that they know it is a possibility, however remote.

Menopause clearly marks the end of the couple's biological ability to have children (unless they have undergone a fertility procedure to preserve some of their embryos), and clients often experience a grief reaction to this phase of life. A grief reaction to menopause is normal—even for those who have not experienced infertility—but the grief reaction for clients who have experienced infertility can be compounded by previous reproductive losses. You can assist your clients during this phase of life by normalizing the experience of grief and facilitating their grief work as you would for any other significant loss that clients might experience (such as the death of a loved one or loss of normal functioning due to illness or trauma).

Using traditional models of grief therapy can be most effective, and supplementing those models with resources—support groups for clients experiencing menopause can be especially effective—and ex-

ercises for couples who have experienced reproductive losses will en-
hance clients' potential for healing. (Journal writing, the integrity
wheel, and the personal loss inventory are examples of exercises that
have been most beneficial for clients in this situation; see Chapter
Eleven.)

Retirement

Retirement, like the death of a loved one and menopause, marks an
official end to a chapter or phase in life. As with all losses and endings,
when individuals choose to stop working there is a natural tendency
to review their past as it relates to the specific ending that is occurring.
When embarking on retirement, individuals are likely to review their
employment experience throughout their working years and to question how they might find other avenues in which to be productive
after retirement. Individuals who have experienced infertility are likely
to be reminded of another time when they questioned their "produc-
tivity" as biological parents (regardless of whether or not they eventually became biological parents). The primary task for these clients
is to accommodate the loss of their identity as employee, professional,
or worker, just as they (ideally) accommodated the loss of their identity as a prospective biological parent when they were experiencing
infertility.

One way you can help your clients accommodate this loss is
through the use of the integrity wheel. As previously discussed, this
exercise can help your clients identify other parts of themselves that
are just as valid as their sense of themselves as a working person. In
this case, the wheel could be used to represent the client's broad range
of interests in order to determine what other arenas could be pursued.
When grief and doubt over the ordeal and the choices made during
the infertility experience resurface upon retirement, clients are challenged to take responsibility for their predicament as they once did
with infertility.

In the same way that your clients had to take responsibility for how
they interacted with professionals, arrived at decisions, and managed
the thoughts and feelings about the infertility experience, so can they
take responsibility for how they manage the experience of retirement.
Ideally, therapy can facilitate the process of grieving over the phase in
life that has ended, and you can encourage these clients to redefine
their sense of themselves as whole and productive individuals.

UNANTICIPATED LIFE EVENTS

Because clients cannot prepare themselves emotionally for unexpected events or disturbing news, these events can intensify clients' experience of resurfacing grief and doubt. Some of the events (and this list is by no means exhaustive) that trigger renewed grief and doubt over the infertility experience are the announcement of new reproductive technologies, unexpected pregnancy, and divorce.

Announcement of New Reproductive Technologies

After clients have been unable to achieve a pregnancy and decide to end fertility treatment, a new reproductive technology may be introduced that is appropriate for the treatment of their condition. When this happens, clients are sometimes prompted to reevaluate their decision to end treatment or experience feelings of disappointment that the technology was not available sooner. When couples choose to reevaluate their decision to end treatment, they must carefully examine their motives for doing so. Sometimes couples feel disappointment about the timing of the new technology's arrival and may experience a reemergence of their grief over their original reproductive losses. This reemergence of grief can be compounded for clients who have biologically progressed beyond their childbearing years and for whom treatment is no longer an option.

The following case illustrates one couple's struggle with the issue of new technology being introduced after they adopted two children and felt that their family was complete. Ben and Liz were in their late thirties when they decided to end infertility treatment and pursue adoption. They were subsequently approved to adopt internationally and later traveled to Russia to adopt a nine-month-old boy and his four-year-old sister. Three years after the adoption was complete, Ben and Liz decided to seek counseling to explore the possibility of reinitiating treatment for their fertility problems.

BEN: Liz and I just heard about a new procedure that we think may enable us to have biological children, and we are trying to decide whether or not to pursue it. We aren't sure about trying it, because we have two children and don't know if it's worth getting back on the roller coaster of treatment to have another child. Sometimes I think if we really wanted another child, we could have adopted again. But then again, this is a chance to have a biological child, and we haven't thought about that possibility for a long time.

LIZ: It probably sounds like we believe that a biological child is somehow better than an adopted one. It's not that. We accept that there are differences between biological and adoptive parenting, and we don't see one as better or worse, just different. It's just that it's really hard to think about letting go of the possibility of a biological child all over again if the treatment doesn't work. I thought we were done with that part of our lives.

THERAPIST: It sounds like you are really struggling between the new possibilities and your old dreams about becoming biological parents. Maybe we could clarify some of the confusion if you could say more about what you believe the advantages and disadvantages of reinitiating treatment would be for you.

LIZ: Well, we know that treatment is a very emotional process and that it can take over your life if you're not careful. We also know we may never have another chance to have a biological child because we are both in our early forties. So we feel like this may be our last chance to try to have biological child, and we don't want to have any regrets about passing up an opportunity like this one.

BEN: I also believe that one of the reasons we ended treatment was because we had exhausted all our possibilities. We wanted to be parents, so we decided to adopt. Adoption has been an incredible experience, but we are wondering if we missed out on something—if maybe our lives would be even better if we had the chance to parent a biological child. I don't know; I guess it all comes down to not wanting to regret any of your decisions. We just don't want to wake up one day and realize that we should have done things differently. So I guess one of the advantages would be knowing that we had tried everything.

THERAPIST: It sounds like you are both experiencing feelings of doubt or anticipating that you might have regrets about missed opportunities, which can be another way of expressing grief. For instance, we often regret not having the chance to say good-bye to a loved who dies, or regret that the loved one can't be with us on special occasions or during times of crisis. In this case, it seems like the increased odds for having a biological child with this new treatment are giving you an opportunity to retrace your steps and offering hope where none existed before. It's like getting the chance to say good-bye ten years after someone has died, but without any guarantees that you will accomplish what you set out to do.

BEN: Exactly! It's giving us hope that we can do it all again, but without feeling so bad this time, because we have a better chance of success with this new treatment. It's kind of crazy when you think about it. Because if it doesn't work, we have been lured back in to the same old game and can wind up feeling the same old way.

LIZ: When you think about it that way, it seems like we are forgetting why we decided to stop treatment in the first place. But the feelings of disappointment have faded. It's like all of a sudden we have the answer that has eluded us, and if we don't grab it we might regret it. I just don't think I can go through that hope, disappointment, hope, disappointment thing again, month after month after month. I guess we need to really try to remember what treatment was like and think about what parenting has been like for us. One was so disappointing and the other has been such a joy. The two are as different as snow and sunshine.

Ben and Liz had to explore the prospects of a new treatment. They wanted to be sure they did not make a hasty decision that they would wind up regretting. At the end of our initial session, we asked Ben and Liz to complete an integrity wheel to clarify all the roles that made up their individual identities. Through our discussion in the following session, both Ben and Liz were able to determine that their roles as "potential biological parents" had been replaced, in terms of significance, by their roles as adoptive parents. They decided not to pursue further treatment and were able to accept that there were advantages and disadvantages to their decision. Both felt, however, that they could move on without experiencing significant regrets about their decision not to pursue additional treatment.

You can assist your clients who are faced with conflicts over reinitiating treatment by helping them to determine if a resurgence of grief is propelling them toward the reinitiation of treatment. New fertility treatment can seem like a panacea for the client's feelings of doubt, sadness, or loss. On further examination, however, clients may discover that treatment cannot alleviate their grief symptoms but instead can have a tendency to exacerbate them. When our clients appear to be reinitiating treatment in response to the resurgence of grief and doubt, we ask them to complete the personal loss inventory (found in Chapter Eleven).

When Ben and Liz filled out the personal loss inventory, we recommended that they focus on their reproductive losses and asked them to include any significant losses they experienced since they discontinued treatment. We asked for information on post-treatment losses because those losses might be a factor in their decision to reinitiate treatment. We also asked Ben and Liz to complete the when to discontinue treatment exercise (Chapter Eleven). This exercise helped them determine the conditions under which they would discontinue treatment should they decide to reinitiate treatment using the new technology. These exercises help us understand our clients' motivation to reinitiate treatment and the extent to which they are willing to pursue it.

Unexpected Pregnancy

Although unexpected pregnancies are uncommon, they do occur. For your clients who have embraced child-free living, unexpected pregnancy can bring excitement, despair, and confusion. Clients who experience the old dream of pregnancy at a time when the dream no longer fits with their lifestyle are in a challenging predicament. The following case illustrates the complications that can arise for couples who view traditional parenting as an obstacle to the new dreams they are pursuing.

Kathy and Hugh embraced a child-free lifestyle after two years of infertility treatment. They had never considered using birth control, as Hugh had a low sperm count and Kathy's uterus had been ravaged by endometriosis. They were told that even if they miraculously conceived, Kathy's uterus would be unable to sustain a pregnancy. Five years after the couple discontinued medical intervention for their infertility, Kathy discovered her pregnancy in the middle of the third month. Both in their mid-thirties, Hugh and Kathy had no idea how to handle an unplanned pregnancy, and sought professional guidance.

KATHY: This is just the worst thing that could have happened for us. Hugh just got a big promotion, and I have just committed to international travel with my new company. I know what all the options are for us, and none of them are appealing.

THERAPIST: What are the options you have already considered?

HUGH: We have considered terminating the pregnancy, placing our child for adoption, and raising this baby. What other options are there?

THERAPIST: Perhaps there are components to each option that have not been explored yet.

KATHY: Like what? Letting someone we know adopt our child so we can have a relationship with him? That would be too confusing for everyone.

HUGH: Terminating the pregnancy is something we could never do. And it has nothing to do with the infertility. Neither one of us could live with ourselves if we had an abortion.

THERAPIST: So what else is there to consider?

KATHY: Raising this baby. I just feel trapped and confused. I had no idea we could be this devastated over having something we once wanted so badly.

THERAPIST: You did not plan for this to happen at this point in your lives. Your confusion is understandable. Don't you think most unanticipated changes have the potential to create confusion?

KATHY: I guess. But I still have no clue as to what we are going to do.

THERAPIST: Have you thought about how you could manage your existing lifestyle while you raise this child?

HUGH: You mean like keep working and hire a nanny?

THERAPIST: That sounds like a possibility. How did you alter your sense of being childless and come to embrace your current lifestyle?

KATHY: By taking the time to look at what we had. We were so afraid of what our lives would be like without kids. We thought we would be lonely and that we wouldn't be understood. We didn't want anyone to pity us. As soon as we stopped living in that grim future, we saw what was right in front of us. Boy, was that a relief.

THERAPIST: Could you use that same approach in this situation?

HUGH: You mean, can we stop thinking about what a mess our lives will be with a child, and just enjoy the pregnancy?

THERAPIST: It sounds like that approach might alleviate some anxiety for you.

KATHY: That is true. Because no matter what we decide, I do have this baby inside of me. I may as well take responsibility for its well-being and experience what is happening.

HUGH: Boy, this is going to take some getting used to.

THERAPIST: It seems to me like you two have already proven your ability to get comfortable with unanticipated circumstances.

Clients who experience an unplanned pregnancy after years of child-free living indeed confront a tremendous challenge. When we support our clients through this crisis, however, we must remember not to get invested in the decision that they ultimately make. What we do invest ourselves in is our clients' ability to draw on skills they have already demonstrated in their infertility crisis; clients can find it difficult to take advantage of these tangible skills in the middle of a crisis. For Kathy and Hugh, their ability to recall how they moved out of a former crisis into acceptance and celebration allowed them to approach their unplanned pregnancy more pragmatically.

Divorce

A divorce formally marks the end of a relationship. Usually, both partners respond to a divorce with grief. Part of the grief stems from disbelief that the divorce is actually occurring, as few people expect to divorce when they marry. Because it is normal for divorcing partners to recall and evaluate the significant experiences that they shared, a couple's experience with infertility may intensify their grief. The divorcing couple may experience a resurgence of the emotions that accompanied the infertility. This resurfacing grief about the infertility, however, will have different implications depending on whether the couple ultimately became biological or adoptive parents or became child-free.

COUPLES WHO BECAME BIOLOGICAL OR ADOPTIVE PARENTS.   Couples often experience profound sadness accompanied by such thoughts as, "After all that we have been through, and now this." This response is particularly common in marriages in which the partners believed that having children would solve their marital problems, as we discussed in Chapter Three. In addition, where infertility once threatened each partner's prospects for becoming a parent, now the divorce promises to challenge each partner's role as a parent, as questions about custody will inevitably arise. Will one parent become the custodial parent, whereas the other has visitation privileges? Will there be a battle for primary custody? Will they pursue joint custody? Because divorce inevitably redefines each partner's parenting role, all possible outcomes to these dilemmas guarantee the reemergence of grief about the infertility experience.

Divorcing couples who have children also may reexperience the sense of powerlessness they felt during the infertility ordeal. This is true particularly in the case of couples who do not part amicably. Any predicament that changes the family system can bring this feeling of powerlessness. A divorce is not only a decision not to remain together: it also causes secondary losses, such as changes in residence, social circles, surnames, financial status, psychological disposition, and parenting responsibilities. Even though couples choose to divorce, the losses not "bargained for" may initially appear too difficult to manage.

You can help these clients by guiding them through several processes. Initially, you can support them while they grieve the end of their marriage, their shared dreams, and their recollections of the infertility ordeal. You can then encourage them to redefine their identities by using journal writing, the integrity wheel, and the personal loss inventory. Finally, you can encourage them to develop interests that do not require the support of a mate, such as pursuing liaisons and friendships with other individuals in similar predicaments.

COUPLES WHO BECAME CHILD-FREE.   Unlike their parenting counterparts, child-free couples who divorce go their separate ways alone. When a relationship has produced no children, divorce represents the dissolution of the entire family. When the partners in the child-free couple evaluate the significant experiences they shared in the marriage, the infertility ordeal is likely to rise to the surface as the catalyst that launched their child-free lifestyle. Partners often ask themselves what they have "to show" for the time and energy invested in the marriage. Child-free living is an obvious and immediate response to this question.

So with the end of the marriage comes the reliving of all the couple's joint pursuits. And with the former pursuit of biological parenting comes the idea of the imagined biological child as a link to the former partner. It seems important to our child-free clients that they establish links to their former mate. They may wish to remain in contact in order to validate the marital experience and to dispel the notion that they are now completely alone when they walk away from their marriage.

When partners who intended to share their entire lives with each other divorce, all the dreams they created together end. You can help your clients regroup and reawaken other dreams by encouraging conversation that focuses on your clients' ability to be fully self-expressed. The integrity wheel can provide concrete direction for which avenues to pursue. Clients also need to explore new possibilities and reconsider their values and beliefs. This exploration should include discussion about the prospective role of a new partner, how things might be different in a new marriage, and the commitment to child-free living in the context of the new life your clients are trying to build.

OTHER PEOPLE'S LACK OF AWARENESS

Clients who choose an alternative to biological parenting, be it traditional or nontraditional parenting, will be subject to the curiosity of others. This curiosity is provoked by any lifestyle choice that appears to lie outside the established norm. Our clients have told us that their chosen lifestyle most often brings out the interest of others at family celebrations and social gatherings. These clients tell us that they are questioned by family and friends with the same frankness with which they were questioned during their infertility experience. Questions from others can trigger grief over the infertility ordeal, whether clients choose traditional parenting or child-free living.

How Insensitivity Affects
Clients Who Are Child-Free

Our clients tell us that even after they have announced their choice to be child-free and included others in their decision, people still ask, "Why don't you have children?" These clients also tell as that complete strangers will ask the same question. People often perceive child-free clients as sad. Others comment that there will be no one to care for the couple in their old age, and wonder how child-free couples find meaning in their lives. These questions and comments usually reflect inquirers' own concerns about how *they* would feel if they were in the same situation. The following case illustrates one couple's difficulty with questions and comments from friends and strangers about their choice to be child-free.

Pamela and Richard initiated therapy after an incident with a neighbor left them feeling confused. The neighbor invited them to a barbecue for families, and told them they were welcome to bring their "children." The couple knew the neighbor was referring to their dogs, Buster and Beasley, but did not understand why the neighbor referred to the dogs as children. Furthermore, Richard and Pamela had no idea why they were so upset by the comment. The couple chose a child-free lifestyle shortly after receiving their infertility diagnosis. They did not pursue medical treatment for the infertility because they were unwilling to invest the financial and emotional resources that treatment required. They decided, instead, to meet their needs to nurture through breeding and showing poodles. Pamela and Richard presented as a dynamic, motivated couple who were particularly insightful.

THERAPIST: You mentioned on the phone that you are uncomfortable with people referring to your dogs as your children.

RICHARD: Yes. They are not children. If we wanted children we would have adopted them. We wanted dogs.

PAMELA: Oh, we understand, people think it is cute. I think they are trying to include us.

RICHARD: But we don't think having children is the only way to be included. After all, we are all people, aren't we?

THERAPIST: I think you are right. So why did your neighbor want to include you in the way that he did?

PAMELA: Maybe because it is the only way *he* can relate to *us*. This way he sees that we all have dependents, in a manner of speaking.

RICHARD: Well, that we do. But his comment made me feel sad, nonetheless. And sometimes I feel sad when a complete stranger just asks if we have kids. I don't get it. This is what we wanted. Why do I feel sad sometimes?

PAMELA: Maybe we feel left out. Well, but we don't. We've talked about that before.

THERAPIST: Maybe you sense that others don't know how to include you. That others view you as left out.

RICHARD: Now that could be it. It isn't that we doubt our decision so much as we know that no matter what we say, there is a good chance that we won't be understood.

PAMELA: Just like no one understood when we chose not to pursue infertility treatment. I felt sad, then. Here we were relieved to be getting on with our lives, and no one understood.

RICHARD: I guess we have always known that we could not make our choice right for other people. At least it is right for us.

THERAPIST: And at least you know you are sad because you want to be understood and not because you doubt your decision.

This couple's grief over being misunderstood when they discontinued their attempts to get pregnant will always be with them. Questions and comments from others might trigger that grief and highlight the difference in the path they have chosen. When clients understand, however, that questions and comments about their lifestyle are usually a reflection of someone else's curiosity, ignorance, or need to relate, they are in a better position to manage their grief and give it expression.

How Insensitivity Affects Clients Who Are Parents

Clients who have experienced infertility and subsequently become parents are often subject to intrusive questioning and insensitive comments about their status as parents. The following are typical questions and comments that clients have reported:

- "Why did you wait so long to have children?" This question is often asked of parents who appear to be outside the "normal" age range for parents with young children.

- "I can't believe you're complaining about the adjustments you have had to make [sleep deprivation, scheduling, a child's inappropriate behavior, lack of time for yourself, financial responsibilities] since you became a parent, after everything you had to go through to be a parent."

- "Are those your children?" This question is frequently asked of parents who adopt children of different racial or ethnic backgrounds, or of parents with children who do not resemble them.

- "So, what do you know about her *real* parents?" This question is posed by people who are curious about birth parents and the information that adoptive parents receive about the birth parents.

- "Well, she obviously didn't get her singing abilities from you. You can't even carry a tune!" (Or her artistic talents, or his predisposition for mathematics, or her temper, or his patience, or anything else that may stand out as a difference between the personalities or inherent talents of the adoptive parents and their child.)

Many of our clients report that they become impatient with such questions and comments and feel that other people expect them to be in a state of perpetual bliss once they do have children. Although these questions can be uncomfortable for parents, most clients report that the questions are especially difficult for their children. Children and teenagers want nothing more than to fit in and to be similar. When other people constantly point out the differences between children and their parents, children feel different or believe that others see them as different.

These kinds of questions remind clients' of their infertility experience, and responding to them often involves acknowledging or referring to that experience. Clients tell us that frequent questioning about their status as parents or the origins of their child can become a constant source of pain for them. We help them deal with their pain by having them express it through journal writing and talking with others who understand their predicament. Clients report that they feel almost forced to continually revisit their emotional response to their previous reproductive losses; for the sake of their emotional well-being they must have consistent outlets for these frustrations.

As we discussed in Chapter Four, we suggest that our clients deal with insensitive questions from family and friends by responding directly and honestly. You might recommend that your clients respond to the questions listed previously in the following ways:

- "Why did you wait so long to have children?"

   "We did what was best for us."

   "We're not in the habit of discussing private matters with others."
- "I can't believe you're complaining . . ."

   "I can! *Raising* kids and *having* kids are two different things!"

   "I am human and get frustrated just like everyone else."
- "Are those your children?"

   "Of course they are!"
- "What do you know about the *real* parents?"

   "We are her *real* parents!"

   "Everything we need to know."
- "She obviously didn't get her talents from you."

   "And we appreciate her for the unique qualities she brings to our lives."

   "Aren't we lucky to have such a diverse family?"

Of course, all of the questions can be met with sarcasm, but we believe that sarcasm makes people angry and defensive and will only create more insensitive questions and comments.

CHANGES IN SEXUAL FUNCTIONING

Changes in sexual functioning are potential stress points for all clients who have experienced infertility. Whether clients are trying to resume normal functioning after infertility treatment, which we discussed at length in Chapter Six, or encountering the changes that occur as a result of aging, which we discuss here, changes in sexual functioning are likely to trigger the grief reaction associated with the infertility experience.

Changes in sexual functioning that occur as a result of aging are likely to trigger feelings of inadequacy that clients may have experienced in the infertility treatment ordeal. The following case conveys the difficulty one couple experienced after forty-six years of marriage.

Greta and Louis sought counseling for the first time just prior to their forty-sixth wedding anniversary. They had one adult biological daughter and were never able to conceive again. It was apparent that the couple never discussed their secondary infertility with each other or with their physicians. They individually assumed that there was nothing they could do about their difficulty with having another child. They had not discussed their sex life, either, until recently, when Louis began experiencing crying spells during their lovemaking. Because they had always enjoyed their sex life, they wanted help understanding what moved Louis to cry so frequently. Greta did not know how to help her husband, and Louis did not understand the source of his behavior.

THERAPIST: Louis, tell me what is happening at the moment you begin to cry.

LOUIS: We are being amorous, and well, I cannot seem to stay where I should stay to finish things for my wife.

THERAPIST: And you were once able to finish things for Greta?

LOUIS: Oh, yes. We have had fun in the bedroom.

THERAPIST: Are you experiencing other changes in your body?

LOUIS: Why sure. I need more sleep these days. In a lot of ways I seem to be moving more slowly.

GRETA: That's true. We are both moving carefully, what with the arthritis and back pain.

THERAPIST: Maybe the crying spells are a reaction to the changes that are happening in your body.

LOUIS: Yes. That must be true. There does seem to be something else, though. I cannot figure it out.

THERAPIST: What else are you aware of when you begin to cry?

LOUIS: I think, sometimes, about Beverly. That is our daughter. I think about how much I love her. How proud I am of her. Is that crazy?

THERAPIST: I would say not. Do you have other children that you think about?

GRETA: Oh, no. He doesn't. We have no other children.

LOUIS: I always felt bad about that.

THERAPIST: You felt bad because you had no other children?

LOUIS: Oh, yes. I always wanted to give Greta an army of children. She was such a good little mother.

THERAPIST: It sounds like you feel responsible for not having had more children.

LOUIS: Oh, I do. What kind of a husband would I be if I did not give my wife the things she wanted?

GRETA: Honey, you have given me everything.

LOUIS: Have I? I have become a crying old fool.

GRETA: Well, you are *my* crying old fool.

THERAPIST: Louis, maybe your crying spells have something to do with your thinking you should have been able to give Greta more children?

LOUIS: Do you think so? Maybe it is because I cannot finish things in the bedroom these days.

THERAPIST: Maybe what is happening in the bedroom these days makes you cry because it reminds you of the days in your bedroom when you tried to give Greta children and it did not happen.

LOUIS: So what do you think? Am I all washed up?

THERAPIST: I suspect Greta will answer that question for you.

GRETA: You have always made me happy, honey. You are not washed up now and you never have been.

From here, we helped this couple begin grieving for the biological children they had not had. As they spoke more with one another about their regrets over not having had a larger family, the frequency of Louis's crying spells decreased. In this case, the spells never diminished entirely, but the couple's understanding of the crying spells relieved their frustrations about them.

Couples who struggle with the changes in their sexual functioning over time find it helpful to know why they are struggling. Gaining self-understanding alleviates the pressure to perform, and they are able to discover new ways in which they can relate to one another sexually.

PARENTING STAGES

Clients who have experienced infertility and who ultimately become parents will face many of the same parenting challenges that all parents face. However, they will also face challenges related to or compounded by their experience with infertility. For instance, all parents are challenged by the need to explain sex and reproduction to their children. But adoptive parents must also explain the connections between reproduction, biological parents, and adoptive parents.

Although the child cannot understand and does not need a detailed explanation of the parenting couple's experience with infertility, explaining the connections between reproduction and biological and adoptive parenting may remind the parenting couple of their experience with infertility and cause them to reexperience grief over their reproductive losses. The challenge to explain sex and reproduction to their child(ren) is compounded by the parenting couple's experience with infertility—they must explain reproduction and simultaneously work through the grief issues that reemerge.

The sections that follow identify specific parenting challenges or stress points in parenting, such as the one we just discussed, that are common to clients who experience infertility and ultimately become parents. Infertility issues are most likely to reemerge when clients encounter stress points that are directly related to their experience with infertility. The most common stress points occur when clients finalize an adoption, educate children about sex and reproduction, answer questions from others, separate from school-age children, and reach the stage when their children are becoming sexually active or bearing children of their own.

When an Adoption Is Finalized

When parents finalize the adoption of a child, they have taken the last legal step in the process of becoming parents through adoption. For many adoptive parents, it is a time of great relief because a finalization legitimizes their emotional and physical claim to their adopted child. However, a finalization can also trigger feelings of sadness and loss, because it also symbolizes the adoptive parents' status as "adoptive" (and therefore not biological) parents. That is not to say that adoptive parents feel as though the child is somehow second best, only that this child has not come into their family through their own conception. Thus, a finalization can serve as a reminder of the adoptive parents' fertility problems, the loss of the potential biological child, and the loss of biological parenting.

Many clients have expressed mixed emotions at the time of the finalization of an adoption, and it is not uncommon for adoptive parents to tell us that they do not understand why they feel "depressed" at a time when they should be feeling "happy." Susan expressed these feelings during a counseling session shortly after she and her husband had finalized their child's adoption:

> I have been crying on and off for about two weeks now, and I cannot figure it out. I feel really depressed and almost let down by the finalization of the adoption. I guess I thought it would give me some kind of ending point, you know, to the infertility. But it hasn't. The finalization just made me think about everything we had to go through to become parents. The losses, the paperwork, the legal risks, and all of the unknowns. I just start crying every time I think about it.

Clearly, Susan was experiencing a reemergence of her grief over her loss of biological parenting. When we encounter clients who are having this type of reaction to a finalization, we try to normalize their response and help them recognize that their response is understandable. Clients often believe that adoption is a means of resolving infertility. It is not. Adoption is a means of parenting, of bringing children into a family. Although parenting through adoption will meet clients' goals to parent, it will neither resolve their reproductive losses nor facilitate their acceptance of those losses. As we have previously stated, we do not believe that infertility can be resolved, but we do know that clients can learn to accept it. Once our clients understand that adoption is not a cure for infertility, we can be assured that they have successfully separated the process of adopting a child from their experience with infertility.

When the Child Begins School

Parents commonly experience a grief reaction when their child reaches school age and begins first grade. They may be suffering from the knowledge that they are no longer the only primary influences in their young child's life. Parents also realize that their child is no longer under their exclusive protection and that the potential for their child to be emotionally or physically hurt by others has gone up significantly. Parents discover that they are no longer privy to all of their child's experiences and that their child is interpreting those experiences without the direct assistance of his parents. Clients who have experienced infertility may find that their grief over their first grader's separation from them is being compounded by their previous parenting losses.

Upon entering first grade, the child's pool of influence expands to include teachers, peers, and other unrelated children for a significant portion of the day. In the first grade, the child undergoes the first formal evaluation of her ability to function outside the home environment. First grade requires the child to complete tasks that help her develop skills for making decisions autonomously, forming peer relationships, and solving problems independently. Unlike day care, preschool, and sometimes kindergarten, first grade is task oriented, and a child can "pass" or "fail" depending on her independent ability to complete the assigned tasks successfully. Parents may therefore grieve not only over the separation of their child from the home and family but also over the child's development of skills that lessen her reliance on her parents, however necessary those skills might be.

Although the grief experienced by these parents is similar to the grief that biological parents may experience when their child starts school, parents who have experienced infertility are experiencing their grief over the potential loss of their child for a second time. The grief is compounded by its familiarity, and parents may have difficulty separating the circumstances of the old grief from the circumstances of the new. They may therefore feel a need to hold on to their child and foster their child's dependency.

It is not unusual for clients who have experienced infertility to become overprotective of their children. Miscarriage, stillbirth, the loss of the potential biological child, the potential loss of parenting—all are losses that clients may experience after a diagnosis of infertility. Parents who have experienced infertility will likely manifest their fear and their need for "control" over subsequent parenting losses through overprotecting their children. Clearly, clients who are overprotective of their children in response to their fear of losing them need to work through their original grief. Parents must also develop skills to cope with their fears. These skills might include becoming adept at self-expression, taking responsibility for their reactions to specific events, and most important, facing their fears by identifying and accepting their emotions. Implementing these skills will promote psychological well-being for these overprotective parents as well as foster their children's independence and growth.

We also work with overprotective clients to help them set boundaries between behaviors that are truly protective and those that may be limiting their children's growth. For instance, we may ask our clients to teach their children problem-solving skills instead of solving their children's problems for them. We also acknowledge, very clearly, that it is painful for parents to watch their children struggle or to see them being hurt by others. However, children must learn to cope with the difficulties that come with peer relationships and their interactions with the external world. We try to emphasize that in the long run, children will be better equipped to deal with problems if their parents teach them how to cope and support them in the efforts to do so, instead of coping for them. We may also ask parents to address the influence that grief over previous losses may be having on their need to protect their children.

When Sex Education Takes Place

As we discussed earlier, educating children about sex and reproduction can trigger a reemergence of infertility issues for our clients. This response can be experienced both by clients who eventually become biological parents and by clients who become adoptive parents. Obviously, discussing sex and reproduction can potentially remind our clients of their experience with infertility, but not all clients will reexperience a significant grief reaction in conjunction with such a discussion.

When clients do experience a significant grief reaction (marked by the reemergence of grief symptoms, such as depression and a sense of profound loss), they will need to readdress their feelings about their reproductive losses. Although some clients may be reexperiencing grief that they did not previously address, many clients will simply be experiencing another stage in the grief process. You can help your clients by letting them know that their reaction is a normal part of grieving and by reemphasizing that the process of accepting losses is just that—a process—and not an event.

When grief reemerges in conjunction with the parents' efforts to educate their child about sex and reproduction, parents may be tempted to delay their child's education about sex in order to avoid their own feelings of sadness and loss. They may also be tempted to delay the discussion in order to avoid sharing adoption information with their child. Although most parents recognize the importance of being honest with their children about their adoptive status, few parents are truly prepared to do so. Parents are unprepared in part because of the complicated nature of sex, reproduction, and adoption, and because of the necessity to explain these subjects at an age-appropriate level.

Therefore, when you are working with parents who are ready to begin or who are struggling with explaining sex and reproduction to their child, you need first to determine that their grief is indeed a factor in their struggle to explain sex and reproduction to their child. After confirming this assessment, explore how they can best address their grief. Second, determine whether their child knows that he is adopted, and if not, examine why they have chosen not to tell him. Third, explore whether they know what information is age appropriate for their child and how to provide that information in an age-appropriate manner. Fourth, determine what resources (books, support groups, articles, videos) are available to help them fill in any gaps in their knowledge.

After you address these points with your clients, you should have a handle on the specific issues that have prevented them from effectively explaining matters of sex and reproduction to their children. You will need to explore each issue and provide concrete tools for managing parents' discomfort. For example, you may want to refer your clients to a grief support group or to other clients who have successfully managed their grief. As we have previously emphasized, when the client's grief over previous reproductive losses is a complicating factor in another life issue, they must first deal with the grief.

When the Child Becomes
Sexually Active or Pregnant

When children whose parents have experienced infertility become sexually active or pregnant, their parents' emotional issues with infertility may resurface. Kae and Don were in their late fifties when their adopted daughter, Page, told them that she and her husband were expecting their first child. Initially, Kae and Don were thrilled, but when Page began to "show," they were struck with overwhelming feelings of resentment and anger. When their relationship with Page began to suffer the effects of their anger, the couple decided to seek counseling.

DON: We adopted Page when she was an infant, and I swear the day she came home with us was the happiest day of our lives. We had been trying to have a baby for ten years and finally decided to adopt. Anyway, we had waited for a child for so long that we didn't believe we would ever get the chance to be parents.

THERAPIST: How much if any of those ten years were spent in fertility treatment?

KAE: Well, we never really did have any formal treatment, we just kept trying to have a baby. We adopted Page through an attorney, so we didn't need to go through any tests or anything. We just had to want to be parents.

DON: We were also looking forward to being grandparents, until Page started to rub it in that she was pregnant.

THERAPIST: How has she done that?

DON: Well, anytime we don't agree with something she says or does or we criticize the way she takes care of herself, she ignores us. I think she's doing it because she thinks we are criticizing out of jealousy. It makes us really resentful of her and, to be honest, pretty angry too.

THERAPIST: Kae, what are your impressions of what is going on in your relationship with Page?

KAE: I feel pretty much the same way. Only I think Page is especially mean to me. She's always sticking out her stomach and saying things like, "Look at how big my baby is getting." You would think that she would be more modest, especially since she knows that it used to make me sad to see other women who were pregnant. But she doesn't seem to care about how we feel.

THERAPIST: Have you tried to talk to Page about how you feel? And what kinds of things does she say to you when you express your concerns? Does she use the word *jealous* or is that more of an impression that you've gotten from her?

DON: No, she doesn't actually say we're jealous, but she does make remarks about Kae not ever being pregnant. That's just one thing though.

We've had several conversations with her, but they don't ever get us anywhere.

THERAPIST: What kinds of things have you talked about?

DON: Well, we've tried asking her if she understands that we are just worried about her health and the health of the baby, but she says we don't understand what it's like to be pregnant and that she knows what she is doing.

KAE: She makes it clear that she doesn't want our advice and that she doesn't want our help. It's like she doesn't need us anymore. She's an adult now and she has her own life, but we're still her parents. Just because we haven't gone through a pregnancy doesn't mean that we don't know anything about it.

THERAPIST: It sounds like you think that Page is misinterpreting your concern for her, and since she doesn't seem to want your advice, you feel as if she doesn't need you anymore.

KAE: That's basically right. There is one more thing, though. Right after Page found out that she was pregnant, she asked us to help her get medical information about her birth parents. She says she just wants to make sure that there isn't anything in her history to be worried about, but I can't help thinking that she is looking for something more.

THERAPIST: What do you think she's looking for?

KAE: Well, she doesn't seem to need us anymore, so maybe having a baby of her own makes her want to know more about the people that had her. Maybe she wants them to be a part of her life now. I don't know, maybe having a baby makes her feel differently about us. Like we're not *really* her parents or something.

THERAPIST: Don, how do you feel about Page looking for information about her birth parents?

DON: Well, I don't know what to think. Sometimes I understand why she would want more information and other times it makes me feel like she doesn't appreciate all we've done for her. We took her in when she was a baby, and we've loved her like our own. I don't think it's right for her to push us away like this.

THERAPIST: It sounds like there are several different things going on right now for both of you. You feel like Page is pushing you away and at the same time she is trying to reconnect with some of her biological history. She is also pregnant, and you believe that she thinks you are jealous of her pregnancy. Do you think it's possible that you may be having some feelings of jealousy or just sadness about never having gone through a pregnancy, but those feelings are not what is leading you to express your concern for Page's health? In other words, that the sadness or jealousy and your concern for Page are two separate issues?

DON: Yes, I think it's possible, when you say the thing about sadness. Because being sad about what you've lost can make you look at other people's happiness and feel sadder. What do you think, Kae?

KAE: Well, I know I really am concerned for Page, because I love her. Not because I'm jealous of her. And she's never really accused us of being jealous, I just think she thinks that because she keeps reminding me that I've never been pregnant. Maybe that's why I'm mad at her, because she just keeps reminding me.

THERAPIST: In addition to her saying that you have never been pregnant, how else does she remind you?

KAE: Well, just looking at her reminds me. Her talking about her birth parents reminds me that she wasn't my child from the beginning, and when she doesn't listen to my advice it reminds me. It reminds me because it makes me feel like I don't have anything useful to offer her.

Kae and Don are struggling with various issues related to their own fertility and to watching their child, who is now an adult, become a parent herself. It is as if they are once again without a child, and being without a child rekindles their feelings about their original fertility losses. In this case, after Don and Kae were able to identify where their feelings of resentment and sadness were coming from, we were able to work through those issues by using their journals, autobiographies, and personal loss inventories. Through these exercises we learned that Kae was feeling useless to her daughter and that both she and Don were feeling alienated from Page. Subsequently, the couple also had to confront their feelings about Page's decision to look for more information about her birth parents and how that decision was also contributing to their grief reaction. (We further explore Kae and Don's concerns about Page's birth parents in the Grief sessions in Chapter Ten.)

THE FERTILITY OF OTHERS

The event most directly related to a client's ordeal with infertility is that of being faced with another's fertility. Some clients reexperience their sadness over the loss of their biological child when they hear of the birth of someone else's baby. The following case illustrates one couple's difficulty with the resurfacing of the self-doubt they experienced throughout their infertility treatment ordeal.

Jack and Johanna sought counseling after attending a baby-naming ceremony for their closest friends. The couple had chosen a child-free lifestyle after six years of infertility treatment and had been child-free for ten years. They were in their early forties and had successful careers and active social lives. The baby-naming ceremony was for a couple who had carried a pregnancy to term after eight years of infertility treatment.

JACK: I have no idea what is going on. We have both been irritable ever since that baby-naming ceremony. We are defensive with each other, and we bicker over things we never bicker over. We accuse each other of doing things that are totally out of character.

JOHANNA: I hate to say it, but he is right. I know it has something to do with our friend's baby. But I do not get it because I am not jealous. We have attended dozens of other baby namings and showers over the years, and I have always felt genuinely happy for the parents.

THERAPIST: Is there anything about this baby that is different from the others?

JACK: You mean like the fact that his parents tried forever to have him? I do not think so. We have known lots of couples who struggled like we did and ended up getting pregnant or adopting.

THERAPIST: Is there anything else about this particular situation that is notable?

JOHANNA: Well, let me see. They are probably our closest friends, wouldn't you say, Jack?

JACK: Definitely. We do everything with them.

THERAPIST: Will you continue to do everything with them now that they have a baby?

JACK: Probably not everything. Still, most things, though.

THERAPIST: People's lives change after they have children, don't they?

JACK: Sure they do. But we do many things with our nieces and nephews. We'll just keep including our friends with the kids like we always have.

JOHANNA: Sure we will. But we'll always go home to our peace and quiet. Now, our friends will have their baby with them all the time.

JACK: So things will be different, I guess.

THERAPIST: Sounds like it.

Jack and Johanna left their first session with some understanding about the implications of change in their social relationship with their friends. Although they knew that their friends would not be as available to them as they once were, the couple did not understand why they continued to bicker with one another. They both reported that their arguments always seemed to go back to the time when they felt so indecisive about which infertility treatments to pursue and for how long.

JOHANNA: Why are we reliving the infertility nightmare after all these years?

THERAPIST: I'm not sure. What are your theories?

JACK: I think it is because we just lost our closest friends to a different lifestyle, one that we chose not to have.

THERAPIST: Sometimes those kinds of losses make us look at ourselves differently.

JOHANNA: What do you mean?

JACK: She means now we feel alone in our lives when we had our friends there with us before.

THERAPIST: Not exactly, Jack. But I think you hit on something there.

JOHANNA: Do you mean it makes us regret our decision?

THERAPIST: Do you regret your decision to be child-free?

JACK: Not at all.

JOHANNA: No, but still, I do wonder.

THERAPIST: What do you wonder about?

JOHANNA: I wonder what would have happened if we had kept trying. . . . Everything would be so different if we had gotten pregnant.

THERAPIST: Yes. It would have been different.

JACK: Is it possible to be happy with a choice and still wonder about the choice you didn't pursue?

THERAPIST: What do you think?

JACK: I guess so. I just hate feeling deficient.

THERAPIST: What do you mean?

JACK: I mean I wish I had some kind of guarantee that our decisions have been the right ones.

Johanna and Jack never came right out and said that the birth of their friends' baby prompted them to review their decision to be child-free, just as they had once struggled with which treatments to pursue during the infertility experience. They did report, however, that their arguing subsided. It is not always necessary for clients to make connections between old and new grief in order to experience relief of problematic symptoms. Clients do need to be supported and validated while they wrestle with what seem to be contradictory feelings. We were able to clarify things for this couple and to expose the reason for the dissension between them through their responses to the decision-making skills inventory (Chapter Eleven). They realized that they were capable of making good decisions despite the absence of guarantees. They were then able to accept their occasional curiosity about what their lives might have looked like had they walked the path not taken.

———

As we have seen in this chapter, there are numerous comments and life events that can awaken clients' dormant grief over the loss of the imagined biological child. Your goal is not to help your clients learn how to *eliminate* their responses to these situations but to help them *manage* their responses. You can help your clients realize that the decisions they make are based on all the variables that are available to them at the time. When they consider discontinuing treatment or consider alternatives to biological parenting, they make choices based on their present situation, the benefits of each choice, and their present point of view. Although these *choices* are made at a particular point in time, we would like our clients to grasp that their *lives* are not fixed in time. It is inevitable that stress points and certain life events demand an examination of former decisions. Whether we prepare our clients for the reemergence of grief or meet them in the middle of an awakened grief response, the therapeutic process can help your clients accommodate all the losses associated with the experience of infertility.

CHAPTER NINE

Regaining a Healthy Identity

You have come here to find what you already have.

—*Buddhist aphorism*

T hroughout this book we have stressed our belief that *successful* infertility treatment, both medical and psychological, must not be defined as treatment that results in parenthood or in psychological resolution of infertility. The key to our clients' healthy adjustment to a diagnosis of infertility lies in how they choose to respond to the diagnosis, not in whether or not they become parents or complete a successful adoption. Unlike the biological capacity to procreate or the results of an IVF procedure, our clients' response to their diagnosis *is* within their control. As therapists working with clients who are experiencing infertility, we can facilitate our clients' healthy adjustment when we empower them to respond to the diagnosis in ways that assist them in integrating the *condition of infertility* into their identities.

There are four key elements in our clients' process of integrating infertility into their identity: (1) recognizing that infertility is a condition and not a definition of self; (2) experiencing grief and accepting that healing comes from allowing themselves to experience the full range of their emotions; (3) knowing that they can proactively manage their responses to infertility; and (4) acknowledging that infertility will forever change their feelings about marriage and parenthood, and their negotiation of the remaining stages of life. As a therapist, your role in facilitating the integration of infertility depends on your understanding of the unique challenges that infertility presents to your clients and augmenting your therapeutic skills to address those challenges. In this chapter, we summarize our model of treatment by discussing how the information in the previous chapters relates to the process of integration. We begin by summarizing the four elements of our clients' process of integration and conclude with a discussion of your role in that process.

RECOGNIZING THAT INFERTILITY IS NOT A DEFINITION OF SELF

In Chapter One, we explained that clients who are experiencing infertility often feel that infertility has consumed their "former" selves. They often define themselves as "infertile" and have disconnected from the other aspects of their identity. In Chapter Three, we examined the ways in which an infertility diagnosis can affect our clients' gender identity and their perceived value as a "biological" male or female. We also described how infertility can compromise our clients' ability to identify with their masculinity or femininity and with the roles they play in their relationships with their life partners. In Chapter Five, we illustrated the effects that infertility can have on our clients' roles as members of society, on their feelings of alienation from the culture at large, and on their role as potential parents.

In each of these discussions we emphasized that it is important for our clients to develop a definition of self that reflects their value as human beings and not one that is dependent on cultural expectations or on their ability or inability to procreate or parent. We further emphasized that in order for our clients to define themselves according to their intrinsic worth, they must stop labeling themselves as "infertile" and integrate the *experience* of infertility into their whole being, along with all other aspects of their identity. In the Infertility and Identity sessions in Chapter Ten, we further explore integrating infertility into our clients' identities; we demonstrate our approach and our strategies for treating individuals and couples experiencing difficulties with integration.

EXPERIENCING GRIEF AND HEALING

In Chapters One and Five we stressed the importance of redefining a healthy adjustment to infertility by changing the focus from *resolution* to *acceptance.* Acceptance is a pivotal point in our treatment model. We define acceptance as our clients' ability to stop resisting the influence of infertility in their lives and to allow themselves to experience the full range of their emotions. We also acknowledged that your clients might naturally resist emotions that are difficult to experience.

In Chapter Three, we illustrated how infertility engenders a sense of widespread loss. We showed how infertility affects our clients' psychosocial (social, physical, psychological, and familial) well-being. In Chapter Five, we discussed the types of reproductive losses and their impact and defined the stages of grief for clients who are experiencing fertility problems. In Chapter Seven, we reviewed the need for clients to grieve the loss of the potential biological child prior to pursuing an alternative to biological parenting. In Chapter Eight, we addressed the potential for the resurgence of grief and doubt throughout our clients' life cycle.

Throughout these chapters we expressed our conviction that grief is an unavoidable outcome of an infertility diagnosis and that grieving is essential to our clients' healthy adjustment. This conviction is based on our work with clients and our observations of clients who seem to be most at peace with their experience with infertility. We have learned that our clients are better able to integrate their experience with infertility into their identity when they see their losses as a part of their life experience as a whole. Clients also seem to do better when they view acceptance not as an absence of grief or sorrow but as a means to integrating all aspects of their selves, including their diagnosis of infertility. For these clients, grief is a natural part of the healing process and is completely compatible with acceptance. In the Grief sessions in Chapter Ten, we further explore grief and healing after a diagnosis of infertility; we demonstrate our approach to healing through grief and outline treatment strategies for individuals and couples who are experiencing infertility-related grief.

BEING PROACTIVE

In Chapter One, we clarified the differences between control and responsibility. We explained that when our clients take responsibility for their reactions to their experience with infertility, they are facilitating their own growth. Conversely, when our clients seek to gain control over their infertility or their ability to procreate, they are seeking to control events and circumstances that are, ultimately, outside their realm of influence. We are convinced that our clients can be empowered when they understand the differences between control and responsibility. Taking responsibility means that clients act proactively and see the ways that they can influence their responses to the challenges that life presents. It does not mean trying to exert control over when, how, and to what degree these challenges occur. By taking this proactive approach to what they can influence—their own responses—and relinquishing control over events they cannot change, clients feel less powerless and overwhelmed. Our job as therapists is to show clients that they have the ability to create and manage their responses to infertility, and that this endeavor leads to their empowerment.

In Chapter Four, we discussed the specific responses our clients may have to a diagnosis of infertility. In Chapter Five, we looked at responses our clients may have in relation to grief; in Chapter Six, responses in relation to sexuality; in Chapter Seven, responses to decisions about pursuing alternatives to biological parenting; and in Chapter Eight, responses to reemerging feelings of grief and doubt. In all of these chapters we showed how to integrate the concept of empowerment—achieved through making choices about how to respond to a diagnosis of infertility—into the treatment strategies that we provided.

When our clients feel empowered to make choices about how they will respond to their infertility diagnosis, the infertility itself becomes less powerful. When our clients reclaim the power they had given to their infertility and thereby influence how the infertility affects their lives, they are acknowledging that the infertility is only one part of the *whole* person who holds the diagnosis. In the Grief, Decision Making, Self-Advocacy, and Financial Planning sessions in Chapter Ten, we further explore empowering clients to make choices about their responses to an infertility diagnosis.

ACCEPTING THAT
INFERTILITY MEANS CHANGE

The final element in clients' process of integration is for them to acknowledge that infertility will forever change their approach to marriage, parenting, and the negotiation of the remaining stages of life.

In Chapters Three and Six, we dealt with the changes that infertility brings about in the marital (or long-term) relationship. We described changes in communication patterns, the focus of the relationship, the sexual relationship, and intimacy. In Chapter Seven, we addressed the changes that infertility precipitates in our clients' paths toward parenting. We explained that whereas some clients may choose to continue to pursue parenting, either nonbiological or with the assistance of a surrogate, others will choose to pursue child-free living. We described the emotional and long-term implications of both choices. In Chapter Eight, we presented the implications that infertility can have for our clients throughout their life. We illustrated how reemerging grief and doubt about the infertility can influence our clients' reactions to life changes, unanticipated events, others' lack of awareness, changes in sexual functioning, the stages of parenting, and the fertility of others.

Our treatment strategies again focus on our clients' ability to choose how they will respond to the changes that infertility brings. When our clients can accept that their lives will be forever altered by an infertility diagnosis and are able to make choices about their responses (instead of resisting those alterations), they have also accepted the infertility as a permanent part of their identity. In the Grief, Infertility and Identity, and Alternatives to Biological Parenting sessions in Chapter Ten, we further explore the life-altering nature of infertility and delineate our strategies for treating clients who are struggling with the implications of infertility in their marriage, their approach to parenting, or in subsequent stages of their lives.

GUIDING CLIENTS TOWARD INTEGRATION

As we stated in the introduction to this book, we believe that our job as therapists is to guide our clients through the challenges that life presents, strengthen their sense of who they are, and help them see that they have the power to determine whether their challenges will shape them or destroy them. We also believe it is our job to empower our clients to respond in ways that will facilitate integrating their infertility experience into their identity and subsequently enrich their life. Our role is that of facilitator: we facilitate healing, acceptance of the condition of infertility, and self-actualization, through unconditional positive regard for our clients.

As discussed in Chapter One, we hinder our clients' self-actualization when we allow our own issues to interfere with or direct the therapeutic process. Conversely, we better help clients who are experiencing infertility when we approach treatment from a knowledgeable, empathic, and objective standpoint.

In Chapter One, we discussed viewing infertility as a condition, encouraging clients to acknowledge their losses, fostering empowerment, and recognizing and treating special concerns. In Chapter Two, we delineated the skills essential to counseling clients who are experiencing infertility. These skills include conveying warmth and compassion, demonstrating empathy, providing reflective listening, remaining silent, avoiding erroneous assumptions, reframing situations, augmenting perspective and context, using metaphors and analogies, using pragmatic problem solving, and providing relevant resources.

Chapters Ten and Eleven provide detailed examples of our approach to treatment. The session plans will assist you in transforming our theories into practice. The exercises in Chapter Eleven are designed to promote your clients' understanding of their experience with infertility. Appendix A contains a list of books and movies, for both you and your clients, that portray our philosophy from a variety of perspectives and in various life circumstances.

Practical Applications

*The last of the human freedoms is the ability to choose
one's attitude in a given set of circumstances.*
—*Adapted from Viktor E. Frankl,*
Man's Search for Meaning

Part Four consists of Chapter Ten, "Session Plans," and Chapter
Eleven, "Exercises." These chapters provide concrete direction
for therapists utilizing our philosophies and approach. They will
help you devise an overall treatment plan for your clients as well as
provide tangible tools that can be directly applied during the therapeutic hour. Each issue and suggested exercise is examined through
specific case samples.

Session Plans

> *I don't like work . . . but I like what is in work—the*
> *chance to find yourself. Your own reality—for yourself,*
> *not for others—which no other man can ever know.*
>
> —*Joseph Conrad,* Heart of Darkness

These twelve sessions focus on assessment (two sessions), grief (two sessions), decision making, addressing special concerns, infertility and identity (two sessions), self-advocacy, financial planning, alternatives to biological parenting, and termination. These sessions also address empowerment, child-free living, the implications of infertility over the life span, common patterns in relationships in which infertility is an issue, the integration of individual and joint needs, the strengthening of relationships, and suggestions for moving forward after medical treatment.

These sessions are designed to be independent of one another so that you can choose the sessions that are most appropriate for your individual client's needs. We devised these session plans with the parameters and requirements of managed care companies and employee assistance programs in mind. We did this so that you can adapt our philosophy for use in as few as three sessions. Thus, each session provides tangible guidance that is not dependent on the client's participation in other sessions in order for an individual session to be beneficial. We provide generic information about the purpose and focus of each session and use a case to demonstrate the application of our strategies for treatment of clients who are experiencing infertility. We also provide suggestions for using the exercises in Chapter Eleven. The exercises are self-explanatory, so clients can complete them in preparation for their initial session or between sessions; they are also useful even after your clients have discontinued therapy with you.

ASSESSMENT

Clients experiencing infertility initiate counseling because they are seeking guidance. These two sessions are spent assessing client history so that we can make appropriate recommendations. The strategies we discuss here are interchangeable within two treatment hours and are therefore presented jointly as sessions one and two. Please note that the strategies can be handled within one session. We mention this because you will not want to spend two hours on assessment issues if your client's managed care company or employee assistance program restricts you to a total of three to six visits.

PURPOSE OF THE SESSIONS

- Discuss decision to seek counseling and direction of the therapeutic process
- Review relationship history
- Discuss motivation for parenting
- Review infertility history

Tim and Leeann

In Chapter Two we introduced Tim and Leeann, who initiated counseling in an attempt to get their old lives back (decision to seek counseling). In our first session we learned that Tim and Leeann had met through mutual friends, dated for two years before they were married, and had been married for nine years (relationship history). We also learned that they had begun their efforts to have biological children during their second year of marriage. In their third year of marriage, Tim and Leeann were told that "everything checked out" for them both, and there were no diagnosable barriers to reproduction. They had tried intermittent medical interventions and reassessments, but had primarily been engaging in scheduled sex for seven years (infertility history). Tim and Leeann were in agreement that their effort to become biological parents just seemed like the thing to do. They both said that they were just about the only ones in their social, familial, and professional circles who did not have children. For Tim and Leeann, having children was simply a function of responsible adulthood and maturity (motivation to parent).

FOCUS OF THE SESSION

- Individual responses to infertility diagnosis
- Joint coping mechanisms
- Cultural, educational, religious, and family views on infertility, and alternatives to biological parenting
- Impact of infertility on the partnership

We did not have the luxury of being able to spend two treatment hours on assessment with Tim and Leeann. We therefore chose to split part of the first session between each partner in order to determine their individual responses to the infertility diagnosis. (Had we had two sessions to spend on assessment, we would have split the second session between Tim and Leeann, and spent the first session gathering relationship and infertility history.) As Leeann demonstrates, our exercise using a pair of glasses with prism lenses (which can be purchased at carnival supply stores) can help us understand how clients view their experience of infertility.

LEEANN: Everyone in my life has their act together. My friends, my sister, my coworkers, just everyone. If I had kids my act would be together, too. It hardly seems fair to me that I am the only one in my circle whose life is such a mess. Why am I so unlucky? (At this point we determined that Leeann's individual response to the infertility experience included feeling separate from others and unlucky.)

THERAPIST: Here. I would like for you to put these on for a minute. (Leeann was handed the prism glasses.) What do you see?

LEEANN: I see multiple images of everything. It's confusing.

THERAPIST: What do you think would happen if I asked you to leave the building and walk across Clayton Road?

LEEANN: I would probably get hurt because I would be unable to judge things normally.

THERAPIST: And what do you think would happen if I asked you to walk around in these glasses all week?

LEEANN: It would be hard, but I would get used to it if I had to.

THERAPIST: And would you be able to walk across Clayton Road without getting hurt by the end of the week?

LEEANN: Probably so.

THERAPIST: What would the world look like to you several months from now if you were still wearing the glasses?

LEEANN: Normal, I imagine. Like I would not even think the prisms were strange because I would have adjusted.

We suggested to Leeann that it is as though she had adjusted to her own unique glasses that make her see the people in her life as included and lucky. We explained that individuals act as though the way they *see* the world is the way the world *is*, as opposed to it being a matter of perception. When Leeann was able to grasp this, she was able to see that just because it looked like everyone else had children and had their act together, it did not make her viewpoint true. Leeann was also able to see that she could hold different perceptions from the one she had held. Leeann realized that there are other glasses, if you will, that she can put on or take off. This new treatment strategy gave Leeann a concrete way in which she could understand her response to the infertility experience and enabled her to see that she was free to choose her response to the experience.

We now share Tim's individual response to the infertility experience so that you can see how accommodating the glasses technique is.

THERAPIST: What is the best way to describe how your life has been affected by your experience with infertility?

TIM: I just feel like our lives are going to be so empty without children.

THERAPIST: It's hard for you to imagine a fulfilled life without them?

TIM: Yes. And I just don't want to be around anyone. I feel like the world and the people in it have nothing to offer. It's all so bleak. (At this point we determined that Tim's individual response to the infertility experience included feeling empty and dreary.)

THERAPIST: I'd like for you to put these on, and bear with me for a minute. (Tim was handed a pair of glasses with yellow-tinted lenses.) Tell me what you see.

TIM: Obviously, everything appears to be yellow. In fact, you need to see a doctor—you don't look so good!

THERAPIST: Is there anything else?

TIM: Well, yes, your white blouse looks stained and old. And the air outside is dirty.

THERAPIST: What would happen if you were to wear these glasses indefinitely?

TIM: I might forget that the air is clear (on most days) and that you are not really sick.

THERAPIST: Like you have forgotten that the world and the people in it have something to offer?

TIM: OK, you got me there.

Through further discussion, Tim was able to see that his view of the world was dismal, and that he responded to the world out of this perception and believed that the world had nothing to offer. Tim realized that he had allowed infertility to skew his perspective.

When we brought Tim and Leeann back together to end the first session jointly, we saw how their individual responses to infertility had created their joint response. When together, both Tim and Leeann spoke in broad generalizations about their predicament (see Chapter Two). They had difficulty allowing different or new information to filter through the different lenses they were each wearing. Furthermore, Tim's and Leeann's individual responses compounded the *reality* of their jointly held belief that their inability to experience biological parenting rendered them complete failures.

We also learned from Tim and Leeann that their motivation to parent (as a function of responsible adulthood and maturity) was an attempt to honor the doctrine of their Catholic religion. They had not considered adoption, but expressed a willingness to discuss it. We were struck by this couple's sense of humor, their openness and willingness to discuss new ideas. They agreed that despite the infertility, the experience with infertility had brought them much closer together.

We could see that Tim and Leeann were close through their nonverbal communication (they frequently winked and smiled at each other in the middle of their sentences) and body language (they sat close to one another and held hands while they were in session together).

EXPLORING OPTIONS

- Review clients' relationship with medical professionals
- Refer to community support groups

Tim and Leeann agreed that they felt comfortable with their infertility specialist, but wondered if the physician was not exasperated with them. The physician had said several years ago that there was not much more that could be done for Tim and Leeann. We recommended that they schedule a consultation with a new physician in order to review their history and assess their prognosis. Tim and Leeann agreed that another medical opinion would help them determine whether to stay on their present course or consider alternatives to biological parenting. We provided the names of several local physicians and referred them to their local chapter of RESOLVE for support and education.

TASKS FOR THE FUTURE

- Journal writing
- Autobiography
- Couples inventory

At the close of our first session we assigned three tasks to Tim and Leeann. We explained that each exercise could benefit them as individuals and as a couple, even if they chose not to schedule additional counseling sessions.

We consider journals private forms of self-expression to be shared at the client's own discretion. However, with clients who pursue infertility counseling, we do ask to review the responses to the autobiography and the couples inventory. This review allows us to determine if there are any special concerns to address before we begin infertility counseling. We ask clients to mail their responses to us before the next scheduled session so that we can read them on our own time. Any information we can derive from our clients about who they are *outside* the therapy hour expedites our ability to guide them *inside* the therapy hour. This practice also helps us to stay within the limited parameters of managed care companies and employee assistance programs. If the answers to these exercises arouse any special concerns, we discuss them at the beginning of the next session.

Journal Writing.   We recommend that clients begin journal writing at the end of our first session because the earlier they become accustomed to exploring their inner selves, the earlier they will be able to verbally express themselves in therapy. Clients who agree to write a journal can benefit from the exercise whether they complete the suggested guidelines we provide (see Chapter Eleven for the complete exercise) or simply record their random thoughts and ideas on a regular basis. After the first session, we usually ask clients to consider at least the questions taken from the section that addresses identity issues.

Autobiography.   Clients who complete their autobiographies benefit from the opportunity to see their present predicament and responses in relation to their past history. Clients can then apply their understanding of their past and present to their future goals and to what they are doing to achieve those goals. After an initial session, we ask clients to complete the section that addresses adult relationships so that they can begin to understand their relationship in the context of their struggle and the choices they have made throughout the infertility ordeal. (The complete autobiography exercise appears in Chapter Eleven.)

Couples Inventory.   Both the process of completing this form and the information clients obtain from it are invaluable for clients experiencing infertility. Couples are able to see their patterns of working together and what things they might be able to do more effectively. You might suggest that your clients begin this inventory by completing the first section, which addresses infertility and its impact on relationships. (The complete couples inventory appears in Chapter Eleven.)

GRIEF

In Chapter Five, we discussed reproductive losses and the stages of grief. We identified five stages of grief that clients who are experiencing infertility might expect to go through: denial and shock; anger and anguish; bargaining; depression, regret, and sadness; and acceptance and integration. As we have emphasized throughout this book, grief over reproductive losses can resurface throughout the client's lifetime, and often does so when the client experiences subsequent losses. In the case of Kae and Don, first introduced in Chapter Eight, their original grief over the loss of the potential biological child resurfaced after they learned that their adopted daughter Page was expecting her first child. In addition to having mixed feelings about Page's pregnancy, Kae and Don were struggling with their daughter's decision to acquire additional information about her birth parents.

As we learned in Chapter Eight, when children are going through developmental stages that ultimately result in redefining the child's or the parents' roles and their relationship to each other, it is not unusual for clients who have experienced infertility to have a grief reaction. In Kae and Don's case, their daughter was about to become a parent, and they felt that she no longer needed them to parent her. They also were concerned because they felt that Page might be trying "to replace them, with her biological parents."

PURPOSE OF THE SESSIONS

- Define issues to be addressed in sessions.
- Obtain a history of clients' reproductive losses using the personal loss inventory (see Chapter Eleven).
- Assess clients' past and present grief coping mechanisms. When you discuss these issues with your clients, ask them to describe any connections that they are aware of between previous and present losses. Connections between losses can include similar responses to the losses; coping mechanisms that have been helpful in dealing with loss; recurring specific themes such as feelings of hopelessness, abandonment, or diminished faith in God or a higher being; or the types of losses your clients have suffered. You will also want to ask about any self-destructive patterns of coping, such as a reliance on alcohol or drugs, withdrawal from significant relationships, suicide attempts, or drastic changes in eating or sleep patterns.
- Educate clients about stages of grief (detailed in Chapter Five).

Kae and Don

During the initial sessions with Kae and Don they decided that they wanted to work on understanding their reaction to Page's decision to search for information on her birth parents. The couple felt as though they were at risk for losing Page to her birth parents, but they also wanted to be supportive of her decision to obtain medical information. In preparation for this session, we asked Don and Kae to provide a history of their reproductive losses by completing a personal loss inventory. We also discussed the stages of grief and their relationship to the infertility experience. Kae and Don could both identify with the second stage of grief, which is marked by anger and anguish: they felt they were losing their child, and their feelings were consistent with this stage of grief.

FOCUS OF THE SESSIONS

- Discuss homework assignments, if applicable
- Discuss differences between having control and making choices about how to respond—accepting responsibility (Chapter One)
- Relate previous losses to current grief reaction
- Share your assessment of past and present coping mechanisms and connections between losses as discussed under Purpose of the Session, above

In the case of Kae and Don, we were working with clients who were past their childbearing years and had already made their decision to parent through adoption. When you are working with clients who are experiencing a grief reaction during the initial stages of the infertility experience, the session focus may also include the tasks listed below. Although these tasks were not applicable to the specific case of Kae and Don, some may also be appropriate for clients who are in the post-childbearing years:

- Discuss cultural attitudes about gender, reproduction, and loss (Chapters Three and Five)
- Develop rituals to mark specific reproductive losses (Chapters One and Eight)
- Discuss impact of grief on sexuality (Chapters Three and Six)

We began the session by reviewing the personal loss inventory and discussing the relationship between the couple's previous reproductive losses and their reaction to Page's decision to search for information on her birth parents. Both Don and Kae indicated on the personal loss inventory that the loss of the potential biological child was one of the most significant losses they had experienced. They also reported that this loss had continued to influence their relationship with Page, and felt that it might be behind their feelings about her pregnancy and her decision to search for information on her birth parents.

THERAPIST: In our last session, you explained that Page's decision to search for information about her birth parents had prompted you to wonder if Page is now wanting her birth parents to be a part of her life and if her having a baby is causing her to feel differently about you. You said you wondered if she felt that you were "not *really* her parents" and that "her decision was causing you to feel like she doesn't appreciate all that you have done for her" and that she is "pushing you away." How have the two of you been coping with your feelings about Page and your role as her parents?

DON: Well, since we filled out the loss inventory we have been doing a lot of talking about why we feel so threatened about Page's decision, and we think it's because we don't know what Page is really looking for.

THERAPIST: How did the loss inventory help you to reach that conclusion?

DON: We just started talking about how hard it was to face the fact that we might not have biological kids, and that led to a discussion about how much we really wanted a child and how in some ways we have always been afraid of losing Page. You know, feeling like she was never really ours, ours alone. In our minds we have always had to share her with her birth parents, but now we might *actually* have to share her.

THERAPIST: So part of your fear is that you will lose Page to her birth parents and part of it comes from feeling like you might not know about all of the reasons that Page is looking for information about them. Do you think that asking Page what she is really looking for might help you to cope with her decision to get additional information on her birth parents?

KAE: Yes, and we have pretty much decided to do that. I think that talking about our feelings with each other has really helped us to sort this out, but that has always worked for us. We still haven't figured out how to approach Page, though, and we were hoping you could help us with that.

THERAPIST: You've said that discussing your feelings with each other has been helpful in the past; what other strategies have you used to deal with problems or issues that you have faced?

KAE: I have always been a list maker, and Don and I have spent many a night at the kitchen table writing down the pros and cons of everything from buying a new house to choosing where we wanted to go on vacation.

DON: You and your lists. Sometimes I think we should make a list of all of the pros and cons of making lists. But seriously, they have been helpful.

THERAPIST: What about sitting down and making a list of all your questions and concerns about Page's decision and then deciding which ones you can deal with by yourselves and which ones you need to talk to Page about?

DON: That might work. We could at least get it all out, and decide what is really important, and figure out a way to talk to Page.

EXPLORING OPTIONS

- Suggest new coping strategies

    Develop coping strategies that will address feelings of powerlessness

    Develop rituals to mark stages of grief or specific losses

    Suggest that clients educate themselves about issues they are dealing with through reading or attending a support group

    Suggest movie titles that may help them reframe their perspective about loss, control, and their responses to the loss

- Offer clients appropriate referrals to community resources

One of the issues we needed to discuss with Kae and Don was their tendency to assign responsibility for their feelings about Page's behaviors *to Page*. As we discussed at length in Chapter One, empowering clients includes teaching them that although they may not have control over the losses they will suffer, they do have choices about how they will respond to their grief. Kae and Don consistently blamed Page for how they felt and were not taking responsibility for their own reactions to Page's behaviors.

Once the couple could accept that they have choices about how they are responding to their grief and thus to Page's pregnancy and decision to search for information, they could reduce some of the stress and anger that was present in their relationship with Page.

THERAPIST: One of the things that I have noticed during our sessions is that you are often able to describe certain behaviors of Page's that you feel have led to your feelings of anger, resentment, and grief. For instance, in our first session I remember you both talking about Page's lack of modesty about her growing stomach and how her lack of modesty made you feel, and how her refusal to take your concerns seriously was making you feel resentful and angry. Do you remember that part of the conversation?

DON: Yes.

KAE: Yes.

THERAPIST: The reason I am bringing that up is that I want to talk a little bit about looking at Page's behavior from a perspective that might make it less hurtful for you. Would you be interested in discussing that?

DON AND KAE: Yes.

THERAPIST: I'm wondering if you have ever thought about your reactions to Page's behaviors as *choices* you are making, instead of looking at her behaviors as the *causes* for your feelings.

DON: I'm not sure what you mean.

THERAPIST: I am saying that you have a choice about how you respond to Page's behaviors. For instance, if Page ignores your suggestions, you can choose to take it personally or you can choose to look at it as a difference in opinion that is not a reflection of her feelings about you but only a reflection of her feelings about the subject you are discussing.

KAE: So are you saying that we may be taking things too personally?

THERAPIST: I'm saying that Page's behaviors may not have anything to do with her feelings about you. It's the same as when you are in a bad mood and you snap at someone. You aren't really mad at that person; your bad mood is just influencing the way you are interacting at that moment.

DON: So you're saying that we might be assuming that Page is trying to hurt us when what she is really doing is expressing her opinion, and it just doesn't happen to agree with ours.

THERAPIST: Yes, and that you are choosing how you let her behaviors influence you.

KAE: I see what you are saying, but sometimes it's hard not to feel hurt by the things she does.

THERAPIST: That is perfectly understandable. Maybe in those situations, when you feel hurt, you could tell Page that you are having difficulty with something that she is doing. That way, you will be choosing to address the problem and giving her an opportunity to clear up any miscommunications.

KAE: It seems like if we did that, we wouldn't always be wondering what it is that she is trying to tell us. I can see it being hard at first, but she is pretty open to talking about things, so it just might work. Don, what do you think?

DON: I think we should add that to our list.

During this session, we gave Don and Kae a referral for a support group for adoptive parents whose children decide to search for their birth parents; we thought a group could help them work through their fear of losing Page and provide them with peer support should Page decide to search for and reunite with her birth parents.

TASKS FOR THE FUTURE

- Integrity wheel (Chapter Eleven)
- Discuss objectives for subsequent sessions if applicable
- Discuss possibility of including other family members in a subsequent session
- Discuss attendance of support group, and assess its value

We ended this session by discussing Kae and Don's goals for future sessions. We also discussed that the purpose of completing the integrity wheel was to help them explore the roles they played in their lives besides mother and father.

DECISION MAKING

As your clients go through the infertility experience, they will be coping with the emotional ramifications of their diagnosis and trying to make choices about their medical treatment, decisions about alternatives to biological parenting, and financial decisions. Because your clients may need to make these life-altering decisions in a time of emotional upheaval, they will probably benefit from a session that provides them with pragmatic tools for effective decision making. As we first discussed in Chapter Two, one of the essential skills of infertility counseling is the facilitation of pragmatic problem solving. Pragmatic problem solving is decision making through the application of pragmatic ideas and solutions to specific circumstances. People can easily apply pragmatic ideas and solutions to a given situation because they are practical, sensible, realistic, and specific. Pragmatic problem-solving skills will help your clients sort through their options and arrive at choices that will bring them closer to their goals.

PURPOSE OF THE SESSION

- Developing decision-making skills
- Modeling the application of decision-making skills to specific issues

Jan and David

We first introduced Jan and David in Chapter Two, in our discussion on pragmatic problem solving. Subsequent to the session described in Chapter Two, Jan and David decided to pursue an adoption. They were overwhelmed by all the information about different types of adoption; they wanted to sort through their alternatives and make a decision about the type of adoption to pursue. At the end of our last session, we asked Jan and David to complete the decision-making skills inventory (Chapter Eleven) for review in the next session.

FOCUS OF THE SESSION

- Review homework, if applicable
- Define the overall goal to be achieved—write down a goal statement
- Define the factors involved in making the decision (time frames, resources, barriers)
- Select an option

We began the session by reviewing the decision-making skills inventory; we asked David and Jan what they learned about themselves from filling out the inventory.

JAN: After we finished answering most of the questions, we got to the last one about patterns in our decision making, and we realized that a lot of our decisions are based on money, on what we can or can't afford to do.

THERAPIST: Could you give me some examples?

JAN: We bought our house because it was in our price range. I mean we liked it, but we wouldn't have chosen it if it had been a more expensive house. We bought our car the same way. I also decided to take a new job because it paid more money. The job was a good move for me professionally, but I wouldn't have taken a pay cut.

DAVID: That's also how we decide where to go on vacation. We look at what we can afford or at what seems to be the best for the money and then decide. It just seems like most of the decisions we make involve money on one level or another.

THERAPIST: So in learning that about yourselves, how does it affect your pursuit of an adoption?

DAVID: We began looking at the brochures and information we've gotten from different agencies and the Internet and comparing the costs of different types of adoption. At this point it looks like we can afford to pursue whatever we want to, but we still want to set some limits. We don't want to get into a situation where we spend a bunch of money and wind up without anything to show for it. Even though money is not the most important thing, we know that we have to be comfortable with the costs and that we don't want to waste the money that we do spend.

THERAPIST: In addition to the financial factors of decisions, what else did you learn from the inventory?

JAN: Well, it really helped us to try to figure out all the factors that we need to consider before making a decision. Question number seven on the inventory—oh, I guess I should say that we decided to use adoption for the question that asked us to name a decision that we needed to make—anyway, question number seven asked us to consider all of the factors that we needed to consider before making the decision, and we looked at time, money of course, and schedules, like if we would need to travel and for time off after the baby comes home. We had a hard time looking at the emotional risks we would be taking and the advantages and disadvantages with each type of adoption because we don't really understand all of that. But overall it was helpful.

THERAPIST: How did you answer the question that asked you to list the desired outcomes of this decision?

DAVID: We put down that we wanted to adopt a healthy baby and that we wanted to try to complete an adoption within the next eighteen to twenty-four months. Do you think that's a reasonable time frame?

THERAPIST: Yes, but it's not realistic for certain types of adoption. For instance, a traditional agency adoption would most likely take at least twenty-four months, and that is being very optimistic. It doesn't mean you couldn't pursue one, but you would need to be comfortable with a two- to five-year time frame.

JAN: It doesn't seem like that is our best choice. David, do you remember what the time frames are for international adoption or private adoptions?

DAVID: It seemed like they could be a lot shorter, so maybe we should focus on those. I think with private adoption, it can happen really fast, but you also take a lot of risks because they can fall through when the birth moms change their minds.

THERAPIST: It sounds like time is an important factor for you. How did you decide on the eighteen- to twenty-four-month time frame?

JAN: We would like to have more than one child, and we are both thirty-five, so we want to try to adopt again and don't want to be well into our forties before we adopt a second child.

THERAPIST: So given the financial and time aspects, what types of adoption seem realistic for you?

JAN: We don't want to take a lot of financial risks, and we want to go pretty quickly, so it seems like a nontraditional agency adoption or an international adoption would work the best.

THERAPIST: Tell me more about the nontraditional adoptions that you are talking about.

DAVID: Well, there are some agencies that do adoptions that are similar to private adoptions only you pay just one fee and they can place a baby with you within a year or a little bit longer. If everything works out.

THERAPIST: What kinds of things have to work out?

JAN: You meet the birth parents while the woman is still pregnant and then work with her or them toward an adoption. If the birth parents change their minds then you have to start again. That's the only thing about it—we aren't sure we are ready to take that kind of an emotional risk.

DAVID: It seems like you could be in for some disappointments. Like what would happen if two or three birth moms changed their minds. It just seems like you could already be pretty attached to the birth mom and to the baby, and that would be really hard.

THERAPIST: In the big picture, how much weight do the emotional risks have in comparison to other factors that are part of the decision?

JAN: They carry a lot of weight. I really don't want to go through that. I have had so many disappointments with the infertility, and I just would rather not go through another series of disappointments.

DAVID: I agree, but we need to find out how often these adoptions fall through and see how big the risks are. I think we also need to find out a little more about the open relationships between birth parents and adoptive parents, because we don't really understand the emotional part of that either.

THERAPIST: What about international adoption? How does that fit with your needs?

JAN: It actually fits pretty well, but we need to find out more about specific programs—for instance, the countries that you can adopt from and specifics about the children's ages and medical problems. But it really does seem like a good option right now.

EXPLORING OPTIONS

- Offer clients potential referrals for implementing the decision
- Further educate clients about implications of the decision through referrals and suggested reading

We concluded the session by discussing resources for more information, and we gave Jan and David copies of brochures for local support groups that assist potential parents in making a decision about the type of adoption that best meets their needs. They were already reading several books on adoption and did not need additional titles at that point. We also gave them an adoption readiness questionnaire and an adoption worksheet (Chapter Eleven) to complete and discuss. We told Jan and David that they could schedule another session to discuss the information they obtained from the referrals and the exercises, or to discuss their final decision, but that they could also complete the exercises on their own and discuss their alternatives with members of the support group. Whatever they decided about another session, David and Jan could use the decision-making skills inventory again to sort through the additional information they received.

TASKS FOR THE FUTURE

- Reassess the decision after clients complete educational tasks, and modify if applicable
- Devise a plan of action to implement the decision

SPECIAL CONCERNS

In Chapter One, we introduced the idea that when special concerns arise during the course of therapy, they will need to be addressed before clients can effectively work through their infertility-related issues. If you do not identify any special concerns that need to be addressed you can skip this session. The following are the most common special concerns we deal with:

- A history of being sexually assaulted
- Addictions (to drugs, alcohol, sex, or gambling)
- Cultural, racial, ethnic, and religious differences between clients and therapists
- Blended or remarried families with children

Your clients' cultural backgrounds, previous traumas and losses, family relationships, and behavior patterns will influence their responses to infertility. For instance, if you are working with a client who was sexually abused as a child, she may need to seek counseling for the sexual abuse before she can address the infertility. Because sexual abuse engenders a sense of powerlessness, as infertility can, an infertility diagnosis may generate new issues about the sexual abuse for the client.

Addiction to alcohol or drugs will influence your clients' choices about how they are responding to and coping with an infertility diagnosis. As therapists, we know that an alcohol or drug addiction can severely impair a client's ability to function in a healthy manner. Therefore, clients may be unable to address their feelings about infertility until they are "clean and sober."

Your being from a different cultural (racial, ethnic, and religious) background than that of your client will also have an impact on the therapeutic process. We recommend that you address these differences in the first session. You can address cultural differences simply by acknowledging that the differences exist. You can also tell your clients that you recognize that values and ideas about reproduction and childbearing may differ depending on someone's religious, racial, and ethnic background. Before making any assumptions about your clients' perspectives on infertility, ask them to share their cultural perspective on infertility and reproduction with you. This way you can avoid making erroneous cultural assumptions about your clients' experiences with infertility.

We have included this latter issue as a special concern because differences in cultural backgrounds may continue to affect the ways in which your clients deal with the infertility experience. If clients are members of a racial, ethnic, or religious minority, you may also need to assist them in their efforts to cope with the "majority." For example, if you are working with clients who are members of a racial minority for which informal adoption is the rule, but they want to adopt through an agency to ensure confidentiality, this session would be useful. You could use this session to discuss the barriers to adoption for racial minorities, to assist your clients in developing strategies to cope with disapproval from family and friends about their decision to pursue a more formal type of adoption, or to educate them about the differences between informal and formal adoption, such as cost, time frames, requirements for legal procedures, levels of openness between them and the birth parents, and the home study process.

Parents in blended or remarried families may need your assistance in dealing with the initial transition of becoming a family, before they can fully address infertility-related issues. When parents in blended families experience infertility and are parenting children from a previous relationship, they must find ways to establish connections to new family members and deal with infertility-related losses. It can be very difficult to establish new relationships during a grief reaction, because grief has a tendency to promote isolation and introspection. Establishing new relationships with a partner's children requires clients to be outer-directed and child-focused, which can be difficult for clients who are suffering the loss of potential biological children.

Addressing special concerns can be as simple as acknowledging cultural differences or as complicated as untangling the relationship between an alcohol addiction, sexual dysfunction, and infertility. The session described here presents a typical example of our approach to working with special concerns.

PURPOSE OF THE SESSION

- Define special concern (usually during assessment sessions)
- Assess appropriateness of referring clients to a support group or another therapist, or set goals to address issue within current therapeutic relationship

Rebecca

We first introduced Rebecca in Chapter Four. We focused there on her changing attitudes about a previous abortion and subsequent fertility problems. Rebecca became pregnant after she was raped by an acquaintance at the age of seventeen. She decided to terminate her pregnancy because she was scared and unprepared to parent a child she conceived through rape. She also felt financially and emotionally unprepared to be a parent. Several years after the abortion, she and her husband were diagnosed with fertility problems. After being diagnosed she began to struggle with her feelings about the abortion, the sexual assault, and the potential loss of biological children. In our first session, Rebecca identified the sexual assault as an issue she felt she needed to work on, so we scheduled additional sessions specifically to address this issue. During the second session with Rebecca, she explained that she felt a renewed sense of powerlessness over her own body and overwhelming guilt about what she perceived as her role in the rape.

FOCUS OF THE SESSION

- Review homework from last session, if applicable.
- Discuss the influence of the special concern on clients' reaction to the infertility diagnosis.
- Assess coping mechanisms.

  Ask clients to describe the ways in which they cope with stress or how they have been managing the particular issue in their life.

  Ask clients about any self-destructive patterns of coping such as a reliance on alcohol or drugs, withdrawal from significant relationships, suicide attempts, or drastic changes in eating or sleep patterns.

If an addiction is the focus of the session, ask clients to give you details about how and when they use the substance or behavior: Do they use it to manage stress in their lives, to repress feelings such as anger, sadness, and loneliness?

Also ask clients whether there are any similarities between their coping mechanisms and the coping mechanisms in their family of origin.

• Make appropriate referral or set goals for treatment as applicable.

We began the session by discussing the homework we had assigned in the first session. Specifically, we had asked Rebecca to start a journal and maintain it daily. Rebecca reported that she had followed through on the homework assignment and had been writing in the journal for at least one hour every day. She said that writing had helped her realize that coping with her feelings of powerlessness about the rape was the most difficult issue for her.

REBECCA: Whenever I go into the doctor's office for an exam or a treatment procedure, I feel like my gynecologist is in control of the lower half of my body. It's like he is violating me every time he examines me. I think it's the loss of control over what is happening to my body; it's weird. I have been having flashbacks about the rape, and I want to stop medical treatment because I think that treatment is causing the flashbacks.

THERAPIST: If treatment is that difficult for you, it may be a good idea to postpone medical treatment until you can feel comfortable again. Flashbacks can be really frightening, and I'm wondering what kinds of things you are doing to deal with them.

REBECCA: I just try to get through them the best I can, but when they are over I feel paranoid about going out in public. I am starting to avoid contact with anyone I don't know well. I just can't believe that this rape is going to keep me from having a baby. I'm really tired of being afraid, and I just want to feel normal. I want to be able to have a baby and I want to be able to forget about the rape.

THERAPIST: It sounds like the flashbacks about the rape are preventing you from doing some of the things you would normally be comfortable doing. Would you say that that is accurate or not?

REBECCA: Yes, it's accurate.

EXPLORING OPTIONS

- Suggest new coping strategies. Much of what you will suggest in the way of coping strategies will depend on the special concern you are dealing with. Attending twelve-step support groups such as Alcoholics Anonymous can be useful for clients with addictions; relaxation techniques may be useful for clients suffering from high levels of anxiety; and, as we have mentioned throughout this book, clients' educating themselves about the issue is always helpful and empowering. They can do this through reading, watching videos, and making contact with others who have had similar experiences.

- Offer clients referrals.

- Discuss advantages and disadvantages of discontinuing medical treatment.

We concluded the session by discussing alternative coping strategies that might help Rebecca deal more effectively with her stress. We practiced relaxation techniques (such as deep breathing and head-to-toe muscle relaxation) and discussed the possibility of Rebecca's going to a female doctor instead of a male. Rebecca thought that going to a female gynecologist might help her relax and minimize the association she was making between the rape and the pelvic examinations. We also reviewed a list of rape recovery support groups; Rebecca chose one that she wanted to attend. We went on to discuss Rebecca's goals for counseling in terms of what she wanted to focus on in therapy.

THERAPIST: In addition to going to the support group, you can come here for individual counseling, or I can give you a referral for a counselor who specializes in rape recovery. It is up to you to decide which one you think would be most beneficial for you. We can work on the infertility issues in conjunction with the rape, or you can focus on the rape and revisit the infertility issues at a later time.

REBECCA: I would like to go to the support group and continue to come here for counseling about the infertility. I really want to continue trying to get pregnant, but I'm not sure I can deal with the demands of medical treatment. I guess I need some support on both sides—for the rape and all of the mixed feelings I have about the infertility.

THERAPIST: I would like you to go to a couple of the support group meetings; we can schedule another session after your second meeting. That way you will have had a chance to get a feel for the support group and we can incorporate some of what you are learning there into the sessions we're having. Once you have seen your new OBGYN and have gone to the support group, we can take another look at your decision about medical treatment. If you would begin thinking about the advantages and disadvantages of continuing the medical treatment, we can discuss it in your next session.

TASKS FOR THE FUTURE

- Evaluate support group
- Assess any changes in functioning and coping
- Give clients when to discontinue treatment questionnaire
- Encourage journal writing
- Provide book or movie titles, and review in next session
- Give clients personal loss inventory

The questionnaire on ending medical treatment (Chapter Eleven) can be adapted to include questions related to the specific concern. The personal loss inventory may help clients remember coping mechanisms that have helped them in the past. Book and movie recommendations should include titles that offer new strategies for coping and healing. Support groups provide peer support, mentors, and a wide range of experiences and coping mechanisms that clients can use in their own recovery process.

INFERTILITY AND IDENTITY

No matter what clients decide about the course of medical treatment for infertility, they must begin integrating infertility into their identity instead of seeing infertility as a definition of self. These two sessions target ways in which clients can move through this process of integration in the therapeutic setting. The strategies we discuss are interchangeable within two treatment hours and are therefore presented jointly.

PURPOSE OF THE SESSIONS

- Integrating infertility into identity
- Strengthening partnership identity
- Increasing self-awareness and self-acceptance
- Accessing and developing coping skills

Rachel and Dean

We originally discussed Rachel and Dean in Chapter Three, and then again in Chapter Six. In Chapter Six, we focused specifically on the impact that infertility had on their sexual relationship. The couple initiated another session, because they felt that they had allowed the infertility ordeal to become the main focus of their marriage. They were still defining themselves as infertile (therefore needing to *integrate the experience into their identity*); anxiety-ridden over their sexual relationship (in need of *strengthening their partnership identity*); unsure of their roles as a man and woman (needing *increased self-awareness and self-acceptance*); and avoiding one another through work (in need of more *effective coping skills*).

FOCUS OF THE SESSION

- Review homework from last session, if applicable
- Assess status of medical treatment
- Begin redefining roles in partnership

Rachel and Dean agreed that they could not discuss their infertility treatment without an argument developing. Both expressed their frustration with the other's lack of understanding for what they were each experiencing. Dean was especially angry with Rachel's inability to accept his long work hours. Both acknowledged that infertility had become the primary difficulty and focus of their marriage.

Review Homework from Last Session.   We had asked Rachel and Dean to complete the when to discontinue treatment questionnaire. They had completed the form, and we discussed their responses. The couple provided a brief history of their treatment experience so that we could assess their present standing in the context of the whole experience, and an update on their present pursuit.

RACHEL: Dean has been doing everything he was told to do. You know, he is wearing the boxer shorts and staying out of the tub at the gym.

DEAN: Yes, and then we did that procedure a couple of times, what was it called?

RACHEL: Intrauterine conception.

THERAPIST: Have you thought about where you would like to go from this point?

RACHEL: Yes, well, uh, sort of. We know what is best, but we are not thrilled about it.

THERAPIST: What have you determined?

DEAN: We are going to do one more procedure and then take a break from all this. Maybe after a little bit we will look into adopting a girl.

Begin Redefining Roles in Partnership.   We then devoted the next part of the session to exploring areas in the partnership that were working. We asked Rachel and Dean to complete the integrity wheel exercise (Chapter Eleven) individually. We then used their individual wheels to help them identify each of the parts that make up their identities.

In the course of the discussion, we asked Rachel and Dean how they might use some of these parts in their efforts to communicate with each other about their infertility issues. They struggled to answer the question, so we provided an example. The example we gave them was related to their roles as friends to others. We explained that their skills in friendships might include listening, providing companionship, and introducing humor when appropriate (we knew that Dean was particularly adept at this). Rachel and Dean each thought of a same-gender friend and then applied their examples to their relationship with one another. Their discussion explored the benefits of talking to each other as friends as opposed to co-partners and co-sufferers in the infertility experience.

From our discussion, it was clear that Rachel's and Dean's behaviors reflected their unspoken expectations of each other. They had shared a traditional marriage in which each expected the other to epitomize the definitions of man and woman. When they were unable to have a biological child, they had to redefine the meanings they had ascribed to their roles as husband and wife. After Rachel and Dean each completed the integrity wheel, they were able to bring the skills they exhibited in their friendships into their marriage, such as the ability to introduce humor and objectivity. In this situation, Rachel and Dean's discussion as marriage partners broadened each person's perspective of the other. They were then ready to redefine the roles they each played in the partnership.

When clients in this situation can step outside their roles as "a person experiencing infertility" and see that their partner is also multifaceted, it enables couples to interact with a previously unattainable level of distance from the grief, frustration, and guilt that can result from the infertility experience. In this session, both Rachel and Dean were able to see that they had allowed the infertility to push aside everything unrelated to their attempts to procreate.

EXPLORING OPTIONS
  • Determine the course of medical treatment
  • Explore alternatives to biological parenting
  • Discuss how to restore sexual functioning

Because Rachel and Dean had already discussed discontinuing medical treatment after one more procedure, we discussed making a commitment to that decision.

THERAPIST: How do you know that you will not be tempted to try again, should this next procedure fail?

DEAN: We do not have any more money, that is how we know!

RACHEL: Plus, I know we cannot go on like this. We really miss the way it used to be, and the longer we go on the way we have, the longer it will take before we find each other again.

THERAPIST: Would you consider yourselves committed to this plan?

DEAN: Definitely.

RACHEL: Yes.

THERAPIST: I think you are committed to this plan in the same way you are committed to your marriage.

RACHEL: That is right. We are going to move on like this because we said we would. Just like we said we would stay with each other for better or for worse.

DEAN: Yes, and we sure have been together through worse, all right.

Explore Alternatives to Biological Parenting.   Despite Dean's prior insistence that he would only consider parenting a female child, we gave the couple an adoption readiness questionnaire. We chose to do this just in case the final treatment procedure did not result in a pregnancy. It is important that clients make rational alternative plans so that they are not left to make emotional decisions in the wake of their grief. We also provided Rachel and Dean with a questionnaire that would help them begin considering child-free living (Chapter Eleven); we were concerned that Dean might never be comfortable parenting a child, of either gender, who was not biologically connected to him.

Restore Sexual Functioning.   Finally, we requested that Rachel and Dean begin to approach their sex lives as separate from their intent to parent biologically. This conversation was difficult because Dean had made it clear that his impotency would not be discussed in the therapy session.

THERAPIST: How would you like to see things change in your sexual relationship?

RACHEL: I just want to go back to the way it was. It is more important to me that I have him, rather than a pregnancy.

DEAN: I would like to be our old selves again, too, but I cannot help but think about the child we do not have.

THERAPIST: That is understandable. Do I remember correctly that you used birth control in the early years of your marriage?

DEAN: Yes, why do you ask?

THERAPIST: Because it seems to me that if you were once able to enjoy sex without the intent to procreate, you might be able to enjoy it again.

DEAN: That sounds good, but now we know we cannot have a baby. Before we had no idea this was the case.

THERAPIST: That is true. But have you considered that because there are only certain times in the month when conception is possible, you could enjoy sex during the days when it would not be possible to conceive even if you were not experiencing infertility?

DEAN: I can't say that I have.

RACHEL: Nor can I. That is an interesting perspective.

THERAPIST: I think it is great that you use the word *perspective,* Rachel. Because I think our perspectives influence all of our behaviors. And if you could begin to view yourselves as sexual beings without regard to conceiving, you just might find one another again.

DEAN: I can actually see how that might work. As long as we don't have sex in the middle of the month, I just might be all right.

In order to help Rachel and Dean function in the ways that we had suggested throughout these sessions, we assigned concrete activities for them to do regardless of whether or not we would see them in therapy again.

TASKS FOR THE FUTURE
- Integrity wheel for the partnership (Chapter Eleven)
- When to discontinue treatment questionnaire
- Child-free living questionnaire
- Adoption readiness questionnaire
- Create-a-date

Integrity Wheel for the Partnership.   Although we asked Rachel and Dean to complete the integrity wheel during our sessions with them, we find it useful for clients to complete one jointly. Instead of thinking of their individual identity issues, the partnership integrity wheel reflects the identity of the relationship. One section will undoubtedly reflect the infertility experience, but the other sections will reflect shared experiences that the couple has lost touch with through their grief. Some of these sections might include laughter, specific activities, friendship, intimacy, and joint hobbies. When couples do this exercise on their own, the experience itself can reestablish a connection that has been absent in the partnership dynamic since the infertility diagnosis.

When to Discontinue Treatment Questionnaire.   Clients should do this exercise on their own so that they have an opportunity to discuss each issue together. The questions are designed to produce concrete answers, enabling clients to make decisions outside the context of therapeutic treatment. By arriving at joint decisions on their own, clients increase their self-determination and sense of empowerment.

Child-Free Living Questionnaire.   Even if you have addressed this exercise with clients during therapy, it is a good idea to provide it to clients whom you do not expect to see again. As couples move through their experience with infertility or along an alternative path to parenting (or both), they can continue to reconsider the ideas the exercise addresses.

Because our model of treatment emphasizes client self-actualization, we give this exercise to clients to educate them about child-free living. Just because child-free living is little considered in our culture does not mean that we are not obligated to present our clients with *all* the alternatives available to them. Requesting that our clients fill out this form is not an endorsement of child-free living, but it is a statement that we honor our clients' right to make informed decisions based on all the information available.

Adoption Readiness Questionnaire. We assign this form for the same reason we assign the child-free living questionnaire. In addition, the questions in this form can help clarify exactly what is expected of an adoptive parent (as in the case of Dean, who felt unable to adopt a male child). If clients honestly assess the issues raised in the questionnaire, they will gain a basic understanding of whether or not they could effectively parent an adopted child. Clients can also determine for themselves whether or not they would experience this path to traditional parenting as rewarding.

Create-a-Date. Regardless of where our clients are in the infertility experience, we ask them to plan special dates with one another, as we discussed in Chapter Six. When clients are able to set aside the kind of time they once did to plan dates with each other, they often experience renewed feelings of excitement, warmth, and comfort. In the case of Rachel and Dean, we anticipated that their dates would help them spark the initial sexual attraction they felt prior to their attempts to get pregnant.

SELF-ADVOCACY

As we have previously stated, many of our clients tell us that they feel a sense of helplessness and powerlessness after they are diagnosed with fertility problems. Their feelings are most often a response to losing a great deal of their influence over the reproductive process. Because reproduction is usually guided by individual choice and is viewed as an inherent option, an infertility diagnosis often leaves our clients feeling as if they have lost control of their own bodies. In response to these common reactions to an infertility diagnosis and subsequent medical treatment, we have designed a session on self-advocacy. This session is appropriate to use with your clients when they feel that they would like to have more influence over the course of medical treatment or the adoption process; be more assertive with medical professionals or family and friends; and be more effective in their efforts to ensure that their needs are met—in their relationships, in the process of gathering information about their options, or in the therapeutic process itself.

PURPOSE OF THE SESSION

• Define issue to be addressed
• Empower clients

Kathleen and James

Kathleen and James decided to seek counseling shortly after they were diagnosed with fertility problems caused by endometriosis. The couple had been to see an infertility specialist; their consultation with her had left them feeling confused and discouraged, and they felt the specialist had ignored their wishes. James and Kathleen reported that they had wanted to talk to the specialist about the possibility of Kathleen's sister Patricia serving as a gestational carrier for their child. A gestational carrier (sometimes referred to as a "hostess uterus") is a person who agrees to be impregnated with and carry to term a fetus conceived through in vitro fertilization (IVF). Because of the endometriosis, Kathleen's chances of carrying a pregnancy were low, but her OBGYN had determined that she was ovulating regularly and that James's sperm count was normal. They had decided not to attempt a pregnancy, as there was a good chance of miscarriage, which they were unwilling to risk. So they decided to try to have a biological child through a donor alternative (using Kathleen's eggs and James's sperm), and Patricia had offered to carry their child to term.

James and Kathleen belong to an HMO that requires them to get a referral for any care provided by a specialist. They had a choice between two approved infertility specialists: the one they had gone to and the one they didn't choose because they had heard so many negative reports about him. James and Kathleen were willing to continue to see the specialist they had spoken to, but they wanted to come up with a plan to ensure that they would not be ignored during their next consultation with her.

FOCUS OF THE SESSION

- Discuss homework assignments, if applicable.
- Discuss the importance of clients' educating themselves about relevant topics.
- Discuss skills that foster empowerment and self-advocacy. See Chapter One for discussion of empowerment. Skills for self-advocacy include seeking education; developing goal statements; anticipating barriers and making plans to address them; restating positions (rather than engaging in an argument, defending an opinion, or allowing the discussion to veer away from the point, clients restate their original position or question and continue to do so until the point is addressed by the person they are talking to); and making lists of topics to be discussed that include specific questions, specific points to be made on each topic, and desired outcomes.
- Review self-advocacy skills and apply them to a specific issue.

Because this was James and Kathleen's first session, we had asked them during the initial phone conversation to begin investigating IVF and the use of a gestational carrier prior to their initial session. We also asked them to do some preliminary research about the medical procedures and to set up another appointment with the infertility specialist they had already seen (because it had taken four weeks to get the first appointment).

THERAPIST: Were you able to schedule another appointment with Dr. Hopkins?

KATHLEEN: Yes, it's two weeks from today. We also went to the library and got some information on IVF and gestational carriers. Well, most of what we found was on surrogacy in general, but it was still very helpful.

JAMES: It's interesting, all this stuff about surrogacy. We really learned a lot and had no idea there were so many different options.

THERAPIST: I asked you to begin reading about IVF and surrogacy because I have found that clients who educate themselves about the procedures they are considering feel more confident when they discuss the procedures with their doctors. I know you said that you tried to talk to Dr. Hopkins about the IVF process, but can you tell me a little bit more about your discussion with her?

KATHLEEN: At first we just told her about the diagnosis, and she said she had already reviewed our chart. Then we told her that we wanted to talk about our options and that we really wanted to try to have a biological child. As soon as we said that she launched into a discussion about treatment for endometriosis. We listened to her and then asked her if she ever worked with couples who wanted to use a surrogate to carry the pregnancy. She told us that that might not be necessary in our case and continued to talk about treatments for endometriosis.

JAMES: So we listened again and then told her that we really didn't want to go through a miscarriage or several miscarriages and that we had been thinking about going with a surrogate. She just looked at us and nodded her head. Then she gave us some brochures about treatment for endometriosis and told us to set up another appointment after we had taken a look at the information. That was it. Consultation over. So we left.

THERAPIST: Did you review the information she gave you?

JAMES: No. We had already seen most of it. Our OBGYN had already discussed all of that with us before we saw Dr. Hopkins. Boy, what a waste of time. She really could not have cared less about what we wanted. She had her agenda and that was that. I was so angry when we left that I wanted to report her to the medical board. But like we told you on the phone, she is our only option. So we just decided to try to figure out a way to work with her. Our insurance won't pay for everything, but it will pay for enough that it is worth it to use an HMO doctor for the procedure.

THERAPIST: It really sounds like the consultation didn't provide you with any new information. That must have been very frustrating for you.

KATHLEEN: It was. It also made us feel like we were barking up the wrong tree. You know, like we should be considering treatment and that having my sister carry the baby was a really dumb idea.

THERAPIST: So now that you have begun to educate yourselves about IVF and surrogacy, how do you feel about it as an option for you?

JAMES: I think we are even more convinced that it is the right choice for us. Patricia, Kathleen's sister, has had two children and hasn't had any problems at all during her pregnancies. We really feel like it would be an incredible experience for all of us. We just want to find out what it is going to take and get started.

THERAPIST: How do you think you could approach Dr. Hopkins and get her to listen to you?

KATHLEEN: I don't. I think she has her plan for us and just isn't willing to consider that we might know what is best for us.

THERAPIST: It might be helpful for you to take Patricia with you to the next appointment. You could introduce her as your sister and the person *who is going to carry your child.* You could also start the conversation by saying that you have already eliminated treatment for endometriosis from your list of options. So, you could say, "The three of us are here to talk to you about IVF and using Patricia as a gestational carrier." That way you would be clearly stating your objectives, and by bringing Patricia you would be demonstrating that you have already taken steps toward achieving your goals. What do you think?

JAMES: Can you just see her face when Patricia walks in with us? She'll probably be wondering who the heck she is. I think it might work, but what do we do if she starts going on about treatment again?

THERAPIST: You can slightly raise your hand and say, "I'm sorry to interrupt you, Dr. Hopkins, but we just aren't interested in pursuing any treatment for the endometriosis. We have decided to . . . ," and explain your position again. That way, you won't be giving her the wrong impression—that you are interested in what she has to say about treatment. She may have misunderstood your willingness to listen to her before as a willingness to consider treatment. You need to be very clear with her, and if she resists, you simply need to stop her and explain your position again and again. Explain until she gets it. What do you think?

KATHLEEN: So we just need to keep restating our position?

THERAPIST: Yes, and it might be helpful if you write it down like a script and practice it before you go in to see her. I know that may seem silly, but it can help. The more prepared you are to advocate for what you want, the more likely it is that you will express it clearly and not get distracted. It is the same with the reading that you're doing. You should be prepared to discuss IVF and surrogacy from an informed perspective. If you understand the terminology involved and the basics of the medical procedure, you won't be intimidated if she starts to use medical jargon. And if you are aware of some of the risks, and understand the odds of success, and the process in general, you will be able to defend your decision if that should become necessary. It is much harder to dismiss someone's point of view when it is obvious that they have done their research. Do you feel like you could do that?

JAMES AND KATHLEEN: Yes.

EXPLORING OPTIONS
- Refer clients to educational resources that will assist them in their efforts to be well informed about their options, medical condition, and so on
- Refer clients to community support group

Kathleen and James agreed that they felt comfortable with this approach to Dr. Hopkins. We provided them with resources for further information on IVF and surrogacy and referred them to a national support organization for people who want to parent with the assistance of a surrogate. We also encouraged them to work out a plan of action if they felt that their next meeting with Dr. Hopkins began to focus on issues that were irrelevant to them. For example, we suggested that they decide on a code word to remind them of their objectives and to take a list of those objectives with them to the meeting. That way they could refer to the list during the meeting and make sure that they met all of their objectives.

TASKS FOR THE FUTURE
- Journal writing
- Couples inventory
- Affirmations

At the end of our session, we assigned three tasks to Kathleen and James. We explained that each exercise could benefit them as individuals and as a couple, even if they chose to schedule additional counseling sessions.

Journal Writing.   In the case of this couple, we might recommend that they use the journal as a means of documenting information that they are given or tracking their progress toward their goals.

Couples Inventory. Both the process of completing this form and the information clients obtain from it are invaluable for clients experiencing infertility. Couples are able to see their patterns of working together and what things they might be able to do more effectively.

Affirmations. Using daily affirmations can be an effective way to begin altering the way in which clients see themselves. They use new, positive language that empowers their behavior despite their experience with infertility. In a sense, affirmations rewrite the old, self-defeating scripts clients once used to define themselves. If clients use them with regularity, affirmations become the natural way in which clients see themselves and their ability to effect change.

FINANCIAL PLANNING

The costs of receiving medical treatment for infertility or pursuing an adoption can require clients to make a complex variety of decisions. Although insurance plans sometimes cover the costs of some types of medical and psychological treatment for infertility, your clients will probably be responsible for a significant portion of the cost of treatment. There are federal and sometimes state tax credits and employer-sponsored programs that may reimburse adoptive parents for some of the costs of an adoption. However, your clients will need to have the financial resources to pay for adoption services up front and then wait for possible reimbursements. The costs of medical treatment and adoption services can run into tens of thousands of dollars, so we are talking about a significant amount of money.

We have developed this session on financial planning so that you can assist your clients in the process of making financial decisions that are within their means, and serve as a troubleshooter for clients who are unable to set reasonable financial boundaries for themselves. You may also need to serve as a mediator between the partners in a relationship when they are at odds with one another about how they will spend their money, and how much of it to spend, in the pursuit of parenting. It is not unusual for us to see clients who have lost perspective on the issues of financial planning while in pursuit of medical interventions that may result in a pregnancy. We also work with a number of clients who seem to be willing to spend an endless amount of money in their pursuit of adoptive parenthood. In both of these kinds of cases, we strongly urge clients to postpone further spending until they have developed a specific and sensible financial plan that will allow them to pursue their quest for parenthood but will not further risk their financial security.

PURPOSE OF THE SESSION
- Financial planning
- Reviewing treatment history and current course of action regarding medical treatment or adoption plan

Jayme and Ryan

Jayme and Ryan had been undergoing treatment for their fertility problems for five years when they decided to pursue an adoption. The couple decided to pursue a private adoption and to continue medical treatment in hopes that they would either get pregnant or successfully complete an adoption. The couple had retained an attorney to provide them with legal guidance about adoption, placed advertisements for potential birth mothers in newspapers in fifteen major cities across the United States, and had an 800 number connected in their home so that potential birth mothers could contact them. The couple had been contacted by half a dozen birth mothers and were currently working with two of them toward a possible adoption.

Jayme and Ryan had participated in two previous counseling sessions, which had focused on assessment and on alternatives to biological parenting. Although we had advised the couple to postpone medical treatment during their pursuit of an adoption, they had decided against postponing further treatment. (We had recommended that they postpone treatment during their pursuit of an adoption because it can be very difficult to prepare emotionally to parent a nonbiological child while going through the emotional and physical cycles of medical treatment. As we have previously discussed, mourning the loss of the potential biological child must come first. Otherwise, the adopted child can easily be seen as a replacement for the potential biological child, and this can limit the adoptive parents' ability to appreciate adopted children for their individual selves.)

After Jayme and Ryan began working with specific birth mothers, they called to schedule an appointment to discuss their finances. They explained that they were confused about how they could make the most of their financial resources. In an attempt to clarify their choices, they had completed our financial planning form (Chapter Eleven), which we had given them at the end of their last session. After they completed the form, Jayme and Ryan realized that they still had some unresolved issues and decided to schedule a session. We asked them to bring the form with them to their appointment.

FOCUS OF THE SESSION

- Review financial planning form
- Assess any spending behaviors that are causes for concern
- Identify any philosophical differences between partners about the intended use of their financial resources
- Set boundaries and goals for the use of financial resources

Jayme and Ryan brought the financial planning form to their appointment, and we began the session by discussing it. The purpose of this form is to provide clients with a concrete means of making a financial plan for treatment or pursuing other parenting alternatives based on their resources, philosophy, and long-range financial goals.

JAYME: I think the biggest surprise for us in filling out the form was finding out exactly how much money we have spent. We tried to use exact figures, and between treatment and the possible adoptions we have spent almost $30,000. That doesn't even include all the money we still need to spend for prenatal care for the birth moms, attorney's fees, an adoption home study, and the GIFT procedure that is scheduled for the end of this month. It also doesn't include the $9,000 or $10,000 that our insurance company has paid.

RYAN: It was the biggest surprise and also the reason for about twenty arguments in the last two weeks.

THERAPIST: What, specifically, have the arguments been about?

RYAN: Mostly about how to spend money. We can't seem to agree on a plan. We just keep going around and around. Jayme wants to stop all medical treatment, and I think we should keep going even though it's expensive. Everyone knows that the more risks you take the more chances you have of succeeding.

THERAPIST: So the differences between you seem to be more about *how* to use your resources or what risks to take.

JAYME: Yes and no. We both know we want to use our resources to become parents; we just can't decide which way, adoption or treatment, has the best chance of success. If we knew that one of the adoptions was going to work out, we could cancel the GIFT procedure. I have a feeling that if we just keep trying with the adoptions, sooner or later it will work out. We have already tried treatment for five years, and it isn't working.

THERAPIST: It certainly does seem that it would be easier to make these choices if you had some kind of a guarantee. However, there isn't any, and I know from our previous discussions that both of you realize that. In a way, your experience reminds me of what it's like to be in a gambling casino.

JAYME: What do you mean?

THERAPIST: Well, when you go to a casino everyone around you is pretty much there for the same reason—to win. In this case winning means to become parents. So if you look at this like gambling, here's what you have. The two of you are placing bets, and right now you have lost more than you have won, moneywise. One of the things that happens when people are gambling is that they begin to believe that the next bet may be the one that "pays off." So they hesitate to walk away from the game because they want to get something back on their investment. Otherwise, all the money they have spent to that point will have been wasted. Besides, all around them they can hear the sounds of other people "hitting the jackpot," and that contributes to their belief that winning really is a possibility. So they keep betting in hopes of breaking even and maybe even coming out a little bit ahead of the game. If they are at a blackjack table, for instance, they might decide to play two hands. Because two hands, as we all know, will increase their chances of winning. But two hands will also cost them more in terms of the initial investment. What I have described is the addictive part of gambling, the part that hooks people and keeps them believing that sooner or later it's going to be their turn. Can you relate to this analogy, and if so, how?

RYAN: I never really thought about it like that. I guess in some ways we have become addicted to the possibility of becoming parents. Is that what you're saying?

THERAPIST: I'm saying that it is easy to lose perspective when you are caught up in this process. The nature of treatment can be addictive.

So can the adoption process, when it becomes a cycle of trying to make up for previous disappointments or losses. You lose sight of the goal—parenting—and begin to focus on beating the odds at any cost.

JAYME: You know, I think that's true for us. We used to talk about what it would be like to be parents, and now we talk about the best way to *invest* our money. It's like we are playing the stock market or something. We have spent tens of thousands of dollars, with no end in sight, and we haven't really given it a second thought. Even with this form we didn't really think about what we were spending; we just started arguing about whose plan had the best chance of success.

RYAN: So what do we do now? We have made all of these commitments, and I'm not sure we even know what we really want.

EXPLORING OPTIONS

- Discuss postponement of current treatment, adoption plans, or both, pending a financial reevaluation
- Discuss alternatives to present course of action
- Discuss additional counseling sessions, if appropriate

Jayme and Ryan decided to end their current pursuit of an adoption and to focus on medical intervention for their fertility problems. Both agreed that a biological child was still very important to them and that adoption had been a safety net for them. We asked them to consult a financial planner before they invested additional resources in treatment. We did this so that they could have a clear picture of their available resources and develop their short- and long-term financial goals. The couple decided that they wanted to continue in counseling because they wanted to take a closer look at how they had arrived at their present perspective about money and risk taking. We scheduled another appointment to discuss the impact of their feelings about the infertility on their approach to decision making.

TASKS FOR THE FUTURE

- Decision-making skills inventory
- Couples inventory
- Support group referral
- Financial planning consultation

We gave Ryan and Jayme the couples inventory and the decision-making skills inventory at the end of this session. They were to complete and return the two forms prior to their next session. We also gave them a referral for a RESOLVE support group in their area so that they could access peer support and guidance about their struggle with infertility.

Couples Inventory.   Both the process of completing this form and the information clients obtain from it are invaluable for clients experiencing infertility. Couples are able to see their patterns of working together and what things they might be able to do more effectively.

Decision-Making Skills Inventory.   The purpose of this exercise is to assess your clients' decision-making skills. The form is designed to access the clients' pragmatic problem-solving skills and to suggest a format for making future decisions. Encourage your clients to use questions six through eleven to make decisions such as those related to treatment, child-free living, adoption, and selecting an alternative to biological parenting.

ALTERNATIVES TO BIOLOGICAL PARENTING

This session is designed to address the alternatives to biological parenting that we introduced to our clients in the Infertility and Identity sessions. Note: this session plan assumes that the client has chosen to turn off of the present path of infertility treatment. We request that our clients attend this session with their forms completed (child-free living questionnaire and adoption readiness questionnaire) so that we can explore the practical aspects of each choice. We also explore the implications for parenting and identity (Chapter Eight) that were not addressed in prior sessions. (Note: sometimes these issues *are* addressed in prior sessions but will take on new relevance once clients are in this phase of counseling.)

PURPOSE OF THE SESSION

- Review child-free living as an alternative
- Review adoption alternatives
- Review medical alternatives to parenting
- Prepare to terminate therapy

Rachel and Dean

We now return to Rachel and Dean, whom we discussed in the Infertility and Identity sessions. Although we had seen them two other times prior to this session, several weeks had passed between each appointment. They had taken the time to explore each alternative to biological parenting, as they had determined that they would undergo just one more procedure with intrauterine conception. Rachel and Dean presented as better connected to one another than they had been in the past, and they were ready to discuss the discontinuation of counseling.

FOCUS OF THE SESSION

- Homework from last session, if applicable
- Practical concerns
- Implications for parenting, if applicable
- Implications for identity

Rachel and Dean brought their completed questionnaires with them, and together we discussed what they had learned from the exercises.

DEAN: It's interesting. After doing the adoption readiness questionnaire I saw that if I was not willing to adopt a little boy I had better not adopt a little girl, either. It had something to do with the question about being able to fully embrace the adopted child's background. I knew I would not be able to do that because I would prefer to pretend that our child was totally ours and that the infertility thing never happened. I guess I don't think I could ever come to think of an adopted child as mine, boy or girl. So I guess we won't be having any children.

THERAPIST: Are you both comfortable with that decision?

RACHEL: I wasn't, at first. Because I could adopt a baby from another planet, if I had the chance. But I see now that Dean would never feel good about it. If we did adopt I would always know that he had done it for me. Somehow the idea of that is wrong. On the surface it seems like a nice thing to do, but I and our child would have this whole life outside of him, and I don't want that. I married *him*, not some unattainable dream.

THERAPIST: What about you, Dean?

DEAN: I wish I could say she's wrong, but she's not. I feel very bad about it. I really wanted to have my own kids. But I am also very lucky because Rachel understands that adoption is a leap I just can't make.

RACHEL: Plus, that child-free living questionnaire really helped me to see that there is a life without parenting biological kids. What really helped me was to go back and answer the questions about our lives before we started trying for kids. We had a great life then; why can't we have a great life again?

THERAPIST: I don't see any reason why you can't. When will you be doing your last medical procedure?

RACHEL: Oh, we already did that a week ago. I'm not waiting on the edge of my seat for the "news" this time, like I was the first two times.

THERAPIST: Why is that?

RACHEL: Because I don't have the happiness of my whole life riding on the outcome of this procedure. Dean and I feel so much better just knowing that all this nonsense is about to end. We even had a date last week on a week night.

THERAPIST: Does that mean you had to come home early from work that day?

DEAN: That's exactly what it means.

THERAPIST: You two have really come a long way. I commend you both for your commitment to one another and your courage to face this experience head on.

DEAN: We are better, aren't we? Where do we go from here?

EXPLORING OPTIONS

- Explore appropriate resources
- Provide referrals to appropriate publications
- Prepare for termination of therapy

At this point in the session, we discussed Dean and Rachel's involvement with RESOLVE and asked if they knew of any other couples who had already embraced child-free living. They said that they had not attended a meeting in a while but knew who to call for referrals when they were ready to do that. We also provided additional information and gave them a list of publications that we thought would be useful (Appendix A).

We then turned the discussion to the termination of therapy. They both requested that we schedule one follow-up session in order to put closure around the treatment. They agreed to call us after learning the results of their last procedure, at which a time they would schedule an appointment.

TASKS FOR THE FUTURE

• Maintaining journals

• Viewing movies

• Reading books

• Gathering questions and all unfinished business for discussion in last session

Maintaining Journals, Viewing Movies, and Reading Books. We requested that Dean and Rachel continue to do the things they had been doing, in order to stay emotionally connected to one another as they moved into the next phase of the infertility experience. We reviewed the benefits of journal writing and provided them with reading and viewing lists (see Appendix A).

Gathering Questions and All Unfinished Business. Before the close of the session, Dean and Rachel agreed to consider issues that they would like to raise in their last session. We explained that we wanted them to walk away from the therapeutic experience knowing exactly what benefited them and what did not and that we did not want them to leave with unresolved issues about the counseling process.

TERMINATION

The purpose of this session is to terminate the therapeutic process effectively.

Dean and Rachel

We continue where we left off with Dean and Rachel. Dean phoned three weeks after their previous session took place to say that he and Rachel wanted to schedule an appointment to update us on the events in their lives.

FOCUS OF THE SESSION

- Complete all unfinished business
- Assess effectiveness of therapeutic process

The couple instantly informed us that Rachel was five weeks pregnant. We noticed that although they were happy about the pregnancy, they were also cautious.

DEAN: I just can't believe it. We were dumbfounded when we got the news. Why, after all these years, it would "take" now—I just don't get it.

RACHEL: I'm so happy I can't stand it. I'm also terrified. It seems too good to be true. You know, if this had happened six months ago, before we started therapy, I would have believed that all my dreams were going to come true.

THERAPIST: And now?

RACHEL: Now I know that this baby is a person and not a dream. The way I feel physically, which by the way is pretty lousy, tells me that I have an awesome responsibility to get real here, to get my head out of the clouds. Through all these years of trying to have a baby, I never really thought about the *baby.* It was always me and Dean I was thinking about: What would our lives be without kids? Will we survive this ordeal? Will we ever get lucky? But now, my exhaustion and nausea have me thinking about this person growing inside me. All I care about now is him or her.

THERAPIST: That's an amazing shift in thinking.

RACHEL: Boy, you're not kidding.

EXPLORING OPTIONS

- Discuss future need for counseling
- Review personal support system
- Review community support groups

Discuss Future Need for Counseling.   Although we were thrown a curve with the news of Rachel's pregnancy, we honored the original agenda of the session, at the couple's request. We let them know that we would always be available for consultation or ongoing counseling.

Review Personal Support System.   We reviewed Rachel and Dean's former way of coping with their frustration as evidenced by their closing
themselves off to each other. Dean stated that he was finished with
seeking refuge in his office and had also begun to reestablish his connections with his college buddies. Rachel told us that she had gone out
with a female friend recently and realized that she had forgotten how
nice it was to be in the company of a friend who knows her well. We
reviewed the warning signs of slipping into isolation (refusing various offers to socialize, increasing work hours needlessly, getting into
petty arguments). We did this to emphasize a former coping mechanism, so that Rachel and Dean would understand that they may be at
risk for adapting this response to other challenging circumstances in
the future.

If you have not already provided your clients with the entire guidelines for journal writing, the termination session is a good time to give
them the section that addresses coping skills. Because coping effectively
with all of life's demands is what will enable clients to remain psychologically healthy, they should be able to assess, on an ongoing basis,
whether they are making the right choices in their coping behaviors.

Review Community Support Groups.   Rachel and Dean admitted that
they were a little nervous about sharing the news of their pregnancy
with the friends they met through RESOLVE. They shared that they
had always met the news of others' pregnancies with mixed emotions
and did not want to cause these feelings in others still struggling with
the inability to have biological children. Rachel and Dean did agree,
however, to explore community support groups for couples who had
gotten pregnant after successful medical intervention for infertility.
We emphasized the need for ongoing support in light of our belief
that a pregnancy does not resolve the infertility experience.

Ongoing support for pregnant couples who have endured years of
infertility treatment is critical, because we have repeatedly heard our
clients say, "Once infertile, always infertile." It is as though clients instinctively know that pregnancy does not cure infertility because nothing can eradicate the experience that brought them to their pregnancy.
As one might expect, this awareness often causes clients to feel insecure.
They fear that the pregnancy is too good to be true and that it is
inevitable that something tragic will happen to the pregnancy. This
insecurity can make it very challenging for couples to enjoy their

pregnancy and the dream they have been hoping would come true. Ideally, support from others who have had the same experience can alleviate some of the couple's anxiety.

TASKS FOR THE FUTURE
- Continue journal writing
- Continue support group involvement
- Continue scheduled dates
- Continue reading and viewing

At the end of our previous session with Rachel and Dean, we stressed the importance of maintaining all the things they had put in place (journal writing, support group involvement, scheduled dates, reading and viewing) that facilitated the healing process. They agreed that without the work they had done as a result of counseling, they would not be facing their future as parents to a biological child with the pragmatic outlook they now possessed.

CHAPTER ELEVEN

Exercises

Tell me, and I'll forget. Show me, and I may not remember.
Involve me, and I'll understand.

—Native American saying

—∿∿—

In our discussion on pragmatism in Chapter Two, we emphasized the importance of providing concrete guidelines for clients in crisis. Often, clients will say, "I know what I want to change in my life, but I don't know how to do it." This chapter contains suggested exercises for your clients to complete when they are dealing with specific issues. These exercises are self-explanatory; clients can complete them in preparation for their initial session or between sessions, or they can use the exercises even after they have discontinued therapy with you.

Homework is an essential part of therapy because it requires clients to independently apply what they have learned during their counseling sessions to practical dilemmas, thus involving clients in their own healing. Through trial and error, clients will discover which concepts work for them and which do not. As the opening epigraph suggests, involvement fosters understanding—in the case of therapy, a greater understanding of self. Homework is a way for clients to gain a greater understanding of themselves outside the therapeutic environment. In this chapter, we provide guidelines for writing journals and autobiographies, creating an integrity wheel, and completing an adoption worksheet. We also include exercises designed to help clients decide when to discontinue medical treatment and consider how to embrace child-free living. Also included are questionnaires for financial assessment and planning; adoption readiness; and inventories for assessing couples' responses to infertility, personal losses, and decision-making skills. We describe the use of affirmations and how to recommend books and movies for your clients.

JOURNALS

In Chapter Five we discussed the importance of clients' keeping a journal to help them work through their grief, and throughout the book we mention specific instances where journal writing can be used. Following are specific guidelines for you to use to help your clients begin journal keeping, and guidelines for clients that you can copy and hand out.

- We recommend that clients purchase a notebook especially for journal writing. It should appeal to the client visually so that it becomes a "place" where they want to spend time.

- Let your clients know that the most important rule in journal writing is to be spontaneous. Stream of consciousness writing or brainstorming are other ways to describe the freedom with which clients should be writing. They should not be concerned with punctuation, neatness, or grammar. The journal is meant to be a safe place where clients can "be" without fear of being judged for their writing style, spelling, or run-on sentences. Most important, in being spontaneous the writer avoids self-judgment.

- Tell your clients that it is also important to be honest. No one but the client will read the journal. Therefore, clients should not be concerned with how another may react to what they have written. Such thoughts as, Am I being too harsh? He would be devastated if he knew I felt this way, or Boy, am I a mess! should not dictate how clients express their thoughts. In fact, questions and comments of this nature can be taken as a good sign that clients are engaging in honest, free expression.

- The last rule to explain to clients is that the journal is a place to reflect, not a place to report. Thus, an entry will not be filled with facts that answer the who, what, where, and when of the day, but rather clients' *feelings, thoughts, and ideas* about what is important to them. It is helpful for clients to take a few moments prior to writing to gather those thoughts. Obviously, they need to take time for journal writing.

We supply some open-ended questions that can provide direction for clients as they begin to express themselves in writing. Eventually, their own voice will emerge. Through writing, and reading their own writing, clients experiencing infertiiity will begin to know themselves in new ways. They will find their own truths. They will trust their own judgments. Ideally, a journal becomes the path by which clients find, in themselves, a friend that generates understanding, acceptance, and hope beyond the experience of infertility.

Journal Guidelines

The following open-ended questions provide specific guidance to help you begin your journal.

TO ADDRESS ISSUES OF SELF-ESTEEM

1. I feel good about myself when I . . .
2. Some of the good things people say about me are that I . . .
3. I want people to think of me as . . .
4. I blame . . . when things aren't going well for me.
5. . . . is/am responsible for how I feel.
6. Ways in which I care for myself are . . .

TO ADDRESS COPING MECHANISMS

Use the list of coping skills to assist you in answering the questions that follow. Consider whether the mechanism is helpful or not.

Daydream	Give up	Withdraw
Try again	Eat	Not eat
Use drugs	Use alcohol	Fight
Take time-out	Yell	Slam doors
Get help	Smoke	Masturbate
Use sex	Go for walk	Role-play

Jog	Pace	Drive
Call friend	Throw tantrum	Minimize
Deny	Exercise	Accept
Act helpless	Meditate	Shop
Draw	Do yoga	Listen to music
Pray	Sing	Dance
Get headache	Tease	Be hyperactive
Cry	Lie	Rock
Get cramps	Clean	Talk it out
Become nauseated	Take shower	Write
Walk away	Laugh	Rearrange room

1. How do I deal with conflicts or problems at home?

2. How do I deal with conflicts at work?

3. How do I deal with conflicts at school?

4. How do I deal with conflicts with friends?

5. Which ways of coping work best for me?

6. Which ways of coping don't work for me?

7. Do I have any behaviors that repeatedly cause problems for me?

8. Are there certain circumstances when this occurs?

9. Does it occur with specific individuals?

10. Does it occur in certain places (work, home, and so on)?

TO ADDRESS CONCEPT OF FAMILY

1. Who are the people in your family of origin? Give their names, ages, and relationship to you.

2. Use three words to describe your family of origin.

3. What do you like most about your family?

4. What is your fondest memory of being with your family?

5. Who are the people currently living in your household? Give their names, ages, and relationship to you.

6. Describe what it is like for you to live with each of these people. Remember to discuss your feelings as opposed to providing a report.

7. Describe what your home life is like, where you live, what your neighborhood is like, and so on.

8. Describe what your responsibilities are at home. What do you most enjoy? Dislike?

9. What do you do in your free time?

TO ADDRESS ISSUES OF SELF-CONCEPT

1. Describe something special you have done or accomplished.

2. Describe how you feel about yourself.

3. List your strengths, your qualities, interests, talents, and so on.

4. Who is most important to you?

5. What is most important to you?

6. Are there any changes you want to make in your life?

7. Discuss your goals, dreams, ambitions, and desires.

REFLECTIONS

1. List six to eight important events in your life. Be sure to include descriptions as well as feelings.

2. For every path you have chosen in life, another path was not taken. Regarding the aforementioned events, answer the following questions: What choices were not made? What did you actively accept or reject? What would your life be like now if . . . ? Create a dialogue between your current self and the self that might have emerged had you taken a different path.

3. Consider your options for the future. Is there anything you are currently doing that you would like to alter? What would it take for you to do that? What is the best thing that could happen to you? What is the worst thing that could happen to you? How committed are you to acting on this? What will your plan of action be? What will you have to give up in order to make this change? Are you willing to venture into new, undiscovered territory? What will support you on your new road?

AUTOBIOGRAPHY

You can use this form alone or in conjunction with the integrity wheel. The purpose of the form is to help clients clarify their values and their perception of themselves, their family, and their spouse. The autobiography is also intended to help clients explore the various roles they have played and still play in their life. It is also an exploration of decision-making and goal-setting methods; an examination of past and present events that have had an impact on the client's life; and a review of past accomplishments, disappointments, and losses. You can use this form or parts of it to obtain background information, either by asking the questions and recording your clients' answers or by asking them to fill it out and return it to you. You can assign the autobiography as homework and ask clients to return it before their next session so that you can review it. This form is useful with clients who are experiencing infertility because it can provide you with perspective on their cultural influences, any patterns of abuse, family dynamics, and marital history.

Writing Your Autobiography

Please answer all of the following questions in full. This form is intended to provide your therapist with background information on you and your family and to give you an opportunity to describe events and people who have had an impact on you throughout your life. Please include details on any significant losses, life changes, or accomplishments that you have experienced. If there is a history of drug or alcohol abuse or other addictive patterns; mental illness; or physical, emotional, or sexual abuse in your or your family's history, and if you are comfortable including that information in your autobiography, please do so.

1. Full name
2. Date of birth
3. Place of birth
4. Physical description (height, weight, hair, eye color)
5. Describe your personality

FAMILY OF ORIGIN

1. Describe your relationships with members of your family of origin. Please include the years that you were growing up, the present quality of relationships, any estranged members, and the quality of your parents' marriage.
2. Who was the family's primary caretaker? Disciplinarian? Decision maker?
3. What types of discipline were used?

4. What values did your parents emphasize?

5. When and why did you separate from your home? How did your family react to your leaving?

6. How did your family handle crisis? Describe a significant crisis and the coping mechanisms of family members. Were crises generally resolved, and if so, how?

7. How was your family perceived by others in the neighborhood or community in which you lived? Did you fit into the family image? If not, how were you different?

EDUCATIONAL EXPERIENCE

1. Describe your academic history, including last grade completed in school, and whether you attended public or private school. If you attended parochial school, what was the religious affiliation?

2. Did you receive any post-graduate education or training? If applicable, what degree did you receive?

3. Describe any extracurricular activities and hobbies and interests you had while you were in school.

4. What was your relationship like with your peers?

5. Describe your overall attitude toward school.

6. Do you continue to socialize with any of your schoolmates? If so, when did you meet, and what is the quality of the current relationship?

WORK HISTORY

1. How are you currently employed? How long have you worked with this employer?

2. What is your current position? What are your job duties?

3. If you have been at this job for less than eighteen months, please describe your previous employment and reason for leaving.

4. How do you feel about your current position?

5. Do you have any future plans to go back to school or to make career changes?

ADULT RELATIONSHIPS

1. Describe your current partner, how you met, and how long you have known each other. If you are not married, describe current

living arrangements. If you are married, describe why and when you decided to marry.

2. Has the relationship changed since you married or began living together? If so, how?

3. How do you and your partner resolve differences, make decisions, and handle stressful situations? What is the quality of your overall communication?

4. How does your family of origin feel about your partner?

5. How do you view this relationship in terms of your and your partner's roles and responsibilities? Do you share similar values? Do you spend time together, apart? How?

6. Describe any previous long-term relationships and marriages. Please include information regarding the length of the relationship, how and when you met, marital status, whether you have children, and if so, who has custody.

CHILDREN

1. Please include physical description, personality description, name, and age.

2. Is he or she a biological or an adopted child?

3. If the child is your biological child, did you experience fertility problems in your attempts to conceive this child?

4. If so, was the pregnancy the result of infertility treatment?

5. If your child is adopted, when did you adopt him or her, and what is the child's country of origin?

RELIGIOUS VIEWS

1. If you are a member of an organized religion, which denomination do you identify with?

2. How do your religious beliefs and practices influence your perspective on your infertility experience?

HOBBIES AND INTERESTS

1. Describe your interests.

2. Describe any volunteer, professional, and religious organizations you belong to.

3. What is your role in those organizations?

COUPLES INVENTORY

The purpose of this exercise is (1) to assess the intensity of the impact of the infertility on each partner in the relationship, (2) to assess the similarities and differences between each partner's perception of the impact of the infertility, and (3) to determine if there are significant discrepancies between how one partner *says* he feels and how the other partner *thinks* he feels. (When discrepancies exist, you should address them so that your clients can clarify them.) You should also be looking for any indications that the infertility has become the primary focus of the relationship—for example, if your clients spend large amounts of their time talking about the infertility and identify infertility as a primary source of conflict in their relationship. If clients are unsure of how to answer a specific question, try giving them examples of possible responses. For instance, if a client does not know how the infertility has affected her self-esteem, you can tell her that infertility often leaves people feeling less confident about themselves, helpless to change their circumstances, as though they do not fit in with their friends or family members who have or are having children, and so on. You should give this questionnaire to clients at the beginning of a session; it should be completed without any discussion between partners.

Couples Inventory

When answering the following questions, please consider any changes in your behavior, changes in your perceptions of the behavior of others, and any significant changes in the intensity or closeness of your relationships with others.

INFERTILITY AND RELATIONSHIPS

1. When does the infertility affect your self-esteem? In what ways?

2. How does it affect your relationships with those you trust the most (identify the type of relationship: friend, sister, and so on)?

3. How do your friends and family feel about your overall reaction to the infertility and its consequences?

4. How does it affect your sexual relationship?

5. How does it affect your feelings about *your* role in that relationship?

INFERTILITY AND LIFE CIRCUMSTANCES

1. How does the infertility affect your social relationships?
2. How does it affect work and school?
3. How does it affect your finances?
4. How does it affect the decisions you make?
5. How does it affect your health?
6. How does it affect your future goals and plans?

INFERTILITY AND THE MARITAL OR LONG-TERM RELATIONSHIP

1. How much time on a given day do you and your partner spend discussing the infertility (including treatment options, finances, reactions of others, stress points, and so on)?
2. What activities do you and your partner enjoy together? How often do you participate in those activities?
3. What are the areas of conflict in your relationship with your partner?
4. How do you and your partner cope with these conflicts?
5. What are the strengths of your relationship with your partner?
6. How do you think your partner feels about the ways in which you are coping with the infertility?
7. How do you feel about the ways in which your partner is coping with the infertility?

PERSONAL LOSS INVENTORY

The purpose of this exercise is to provide both you and the client with insight into the client's history of loss, how past losses may be affecting the client's perspective on his reproductive losses, how the client copes with loss over time, and how the client has integrated previous losses into his present identity. You can ask clients to focus on their reproductive losses when they are filling out this form or to address loss in general.

When you review this form you should be looking for connections between past and present losses and any impact that previous losses may be having on your client's experience with infertility. When you discuss this form with your clients, you can also ask them to describe any connections that they are aware of between previous and present losses. Connections between losses can include similar responses to the losses; coping mechanisms that have been helpful in dealing with loss; recurring specific themes such as feelings of hopelessness, abandonment, or diminished faith in God or a higher being; or the types of losses your clients have suffered—for example, many of their losses may be related to infertility, or the loss of loved ones, or the loss of financial security.

Personal Loss Inventory

1. Specify three life-altering losses that you have experienced in your life. Do not limit your description to the death of a loved one: life-altering losses may include the loss of personal belongings, aspirations, or dreams; the loss of a person through separation (as in divorce or the ending of a relationship); and losses associated with violence or trauma (for example, loss of normal sexual development because of sexual abuse, loss of security because you were victimized by crime, or loss of normal functioning because of an accident or injury). Briefly describe how these losses affected your life, relationships, or functioning.

2. Choose one of these losses and briefly describe how you addressed the impact of the loss, what you feel you learned as a result of the loss, and what, if any, effects this loss continues to have on you.

DECISION-MAKING SKILLS INVENTORY

The purpose of this exercise is to assess your client's decision-making skills; it is intended to be given as a homework assignment. This form is designed to access the client's pragmatic problem-solving skills and to suggest a format for making future decisions. Encourage your clients to use questions six through eleven to make decisions such as those related to treatment, child-free living, adoption, and selecting an alternative to biological parenting. You can simply tell clients that this form is designed to help them identify their patterns of decision making and that you will discuss their answers to the questions during the following session.

Decision-Making Skills Inventory

1. Describe the most significant decision you have ever made. What, specifically, made this decision so significant? (For instance, did it result in major life changes, a large financial commitment, or to the dissolution of an important relationship?)

2. What did you feel were the advantages and disadvantages of this decision at the time you made it?

3. In the long run, what have the advantages and disadvantages of this decision been?

4. What alternatives did you have? Which ones did you consider before making this decision?

5. Are there any types of decisions that you make on a regular basis (for instance, decisions about family, career, finances, or lifestyle)? What are they? What factors go into making these decisions? Do you generally find that your decisions about these issues result in the intended outcomes?

6. Describe a decision you need to make.

7. List all the factors (time, money, geography, schedules, emotional impact, enlisting the cooperation of others, your spouse's perspective, and the like) that you need to consider before making this decision.

8. List all the options you have to choose from. (For instance, if you are trying to decide whether or not to sell your house, your options might include renting it, remodeling it, or refinancing your loan to lower the payments.)

9. What are the advantages and disadvantages of each option? (Itemize for each option.)

10. What are the desired outcomes of this decision?

11. What steps will you need to take to ensure those outcomes? (Itemize each step.)

12. Do you see any patterns in the ways that you make decisions? If so, what are they? Do you think these patterns contribute to or detract from your ability to achieve your goals? How, if at all, would you change the ways in which you make decisions?

INTEGRITY WHEEL

The integrity wheel is a tool created to help clients see all aspects of their identity in relationship to their entire being. You will guide clients through this exercise in the therapy session. Once clients have used the tool in session, they can be given blank charts to use on their own for other entities, such as the identity of their intimate relationship.

The integrity wheel is simply a circle divided into numerous sections—a pie chart. Ask your clients to put their name at the top of the wheel and let them know that this chart will represent them when it is complete. Then request that they fill in each section with a word or statement that represents one aspect of their identity.

Because many clients are unclear about what an aspect of their identity is, you can tell them that a part of their identity is something central to their being that makes them specifically who they are, such as their race, religion, and gender. After you give them these "freebies" you can ask them to define themselves further. The wheels usually depict roles, such as wife, sister, and friend. The wheel may also reveal a profession, interest, or hobby. Regarding the experience of infertility, we hope to see "prospective parent" or "child-free adult" as opposed to "infertile person," but nonetheless, the goal for the client is to be able to see that the "infertility" slice is only one aspect of her identity.

After your client has completed the integrity wheel, hand him a highlighter and ask him to mark through all of the sections that represent areas in his life that he feels are not fully self-expressed. It is normal for everyone to have numerous highlighted areas. You can tell this to the client in order to let him know that highlighted areas do not indicate that something is wrong but rather that he is not honoring all aspects of his true self. Explain that the lack of integration (meaning that the whole self is not fully expressed) is the reason the client is suffering, *and not because he does not have children.* (The figure illustrates a completed chart. You can create a blank wheel for your clients to use.)

Next, look at the areas in your client's life that appear to have simple solutions to increase self-expression. One client we know highlighted a section labeled "artist" and explained that she was not fully self-expressed in her art work because she had to clean up her supplies after each painting session. She said that one block of time was not enough time to create a painting. After working on the integrity wheel, she decided to create a space in her basement that would give

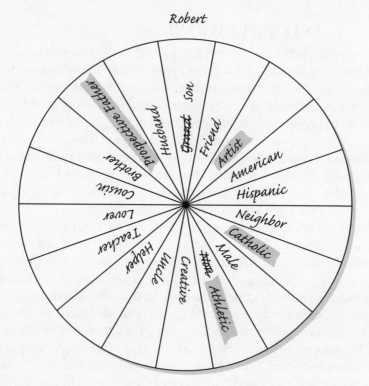

her the room to paint and leave her unfinished work untouched. Just the possibility of honoring her need to paint liberated this client from her despair regarding her lack of fulfillment as an artist. (We use an example that is unrelated to infertility to emphasize that clients are not their diagnosis of infertility. Also, it is often easier for clients to tackle these unrelated areas first and then move on to the more threatening identity issue of "infertile.")

Because the pie slice labeled "infertile" or "prospective parent" is always highlighted, you can explore how this particular aspect of the client's identity might be fully expressed without the experience of biological parenting. Usually, clients begin to explore other definitions of parenting and share information with us that they have not mentioned before. Some of this information might include their roles as godparents to a friend's child, or opportunities they have to take nephews and nieces on special outings and vacations. It is important that you emphasize that these other avenues for parenting are not to be viewed as *substitutes* for the biological parenting the client hopes to experience. Rather, these avenues are redefinitions of ways in which to meet your client's need to be nurturing and loving in adult-child relationships. In addition, your clients may want to redefine the concept of permanency in child rearing. They might consider the many avenues of meeting the need to parent that may be temporary or intermittent, such as in foster parenting and the Big Brother and Big Sister programs.

Through redefining ways in which parenting can be expressed, your clients create options for their self-expression and are no longer confined to the narrow definition of biological parenting. Thus their sense of well-being is no longer contingent on whether or not they achieve a pregnancy and conquer infertility.

FINANCIAL ASSESSMENT AND PLANNING

The purpose of this questionnaire is to provide clients with a concrete means of making a financial plan for treatment or for pursuing other parenting alternatives based on their resources, philosophy, and long-range financial goals. The questions are designed to illuminate and clarify any philosophical differences that clients may have with each other about their financial plans for treatment, and to raise questions that clients may not have considered before. Because clients will need to review their financial records to complete this form, it is best used as a homework assignment.

Financial Assessment and Planning Form

The purpose of this form is to provide you with a concrete means of making a financial plan for treatment or for pursuing other parenting alternatives based on your financial resources, philosophy about money, and long-range financial goals. Before completing this form, you may find it helpful to gather financial documents and information on insurance coverage, available reimbursements for adoption (including federal and state tax credits, employer benefits, and subsidies for children with special needs who are adopted domestically). If there are questions that you and your partner disagree on, leave them blank and reconsider them after completing the financial philosophy section of this exercise.

FINANCIAL RESOURCES

1. Record your total investment in diagnostic and treatment procedures, to date.

2. List the cost, per attempt, of medical procedures and/or adoption processes you are considering; use a three-column format with the following headings: *Procedure, Cost,* and *Recommended Number of Attempts.*

3. Record the total cost of pending procedures to which you have committed.

4. Record the estimated total of available financial resources (total should include all resources, not just those available for medical treatment or adoption).

5. Record the estimated total of financial resources you are willing to commit to treatment.

6. If adoption is an option, record the estimated total financial resources you are willing to commit to pursuing an adoption.

7. Record your remaining financial resources.

8. Over the next two years, what is the estimated total of financial resources that may become available?

9. What portion of these resources are you willing to commit to either treatment or adoption?

10. How much debt, if any, are you willing to incur for treatment or adoption?

FINANCIAL PHILOSOPHY

1. Was the decision-making process for answering the previous questions similar to the process you would normally engage in when making financial decisions? If not, how was it different?

2. Were there any significant disagreements between you and your partner about any of the resource questions? If yes, summarize the differences between your perspectives, and list possible compromises.

3. If you were willing to incur debt to finance either treatment or an adoption, what is your plan for repaying that debt? Be specific (list amounts of payments, source of funds, and time frames for repayment).

4. If you are considering adoption, have you considered the financial ramifications of an adoption that falls through? What financial options will you have to pursue a second adoption? (To answer this question, you may need to contact several adoption agencies to obtain estimates of the pre-placement or pre-finalization financial requirements, such as prenatal care costs, travel, legal fees, and home study fees.)

5. Have you considered the cost of preparing your home for a child, the costs involved for multiple births (such as the additional medical costs for premature births, which are more common with multiple-fetus pregnancies), insurance costs, costs of meeting the child's basic needs, and child-care expenses?

6. If the financial decisions you have made will put a strain on your budget, have you discussed how this strain might affect your marriage and your parenting? Explain.

7. If you are unable to set realistic limits on the amounts that you are willing to spend, or if you find yourselves committing thousands of dollars to high-risk, low-probability procedures, have you considered the possibility that you may need to take a break from treatment? (Sometimes taking a break from treatment can restore objectivity and renew your capacity to make decisions from a more balanced perspective.) How do you and your partner feel about taking a break from treatment?

8. Using your answers to the previous questions, develop a goal statement regarding finances and treatment or adoption. Include strategies for accomplishing this goal.

WHEN TO DISCONTINUE TREATMENT

The following exercise is designed to help clients determine the direction and course of treatment. The most common reason for the discontinuation of medical treatment is the achievement of a pregnancy. Some clients, however, drift in treatment without a long-term plan. These clients are at risk for feeling powerless. The following questions are designed to help your clients determine for themselves when enough is enough. Remember, the answers themselves are not as important as your clients' ability to make a decision and commit to that decision.

When to Discontinue Treatment

1. How much money are you willing to spend on infertility treatment?

    • Are you willing to spend your savings?

    • Are you willing to incur debt?

    • Are you willing to jeopardize your medical insurability?

2. How long are you willing to undergo treatment?

    • For how many months or years will you endure physical discomfort?

    • For how many months or years will you forfeit your privacy?

    • For how many months or years will you compromise your sexual freedom?

    • For how many months or years will you compromise your psychological and emotional well-being?

3. What will it take for you to know, regardless of new technologies, that you are finished with all attempts to conceive through medical intervention?

    • You must achieve a pregnancy and carry to full term.

    • Your physician tells you there is nothing more that can be done.

    • Your partner tells you that the relationship is at risk.

    • You have used all of your financial resources.

    • You have (or your partner has) experienced menopause.

    • You decide to consider alternatives to biological parenting.

    • You realize that your life has become consumed by infertility and that you want more than this for yourself and your partner.

CONSIDERING CHILD-FREE LIVING

Child-free living is a rarely considered option for clients who are experiencing no success with medical intervention for infertility. Clients come to consider a child-free lifestyle for a multitude of reasons. The critical feature of child-free living is that clients *choose* to be child-free rather than remain without children in resignation that they are unable to have biological children. Becoming child-free is a process by

which couples intentionally discontinue infertility treatment procedures, consider the use of birth control (depending on the infertility
diagnosis), and embrace all that is already working in their lives. Use
the following questionnaire to help your clients consider child-free
living as an alternative to biological parenting. If the responses to the
questions indicate an openness to child-free living, your client has
probably done a fair amount of grieving over the loss of the biological
child and is ready to move into the acceptance phase of their experience with infertility. If the responses evoke sorrow, anger, or bewilderment, you may want to consider the use of the when to discontinue
treatment exercise.

Considering Child-Free Living

1. Prior to your decision to have biological children, what made
   you happy?
   - What were your interests?
   - What activities did you participate in?
   - What were your hobbies?
   - What did you share as a couple?
2. What was your motivation to have children?
   - Why did you want children?
   - Did you want an opportunity to nurture?
     - What other outlets can you pursue in order to fulfill your
       need to nurture?
     - Can any of the following roles and activities meet your
       need to nurture?
       - Big Brother or Big Sister programs
       - Foster parenting
       - Girl Scout or Boy Scout leadership
       - Little League coaching
       - Temple, church, or synagogue youth group leadership
       - Animal care
       - Gardening
       - Volunteering at a day care or residential treatment facility

3. Were you hoping to contribute something tangible to the world?
   - How else can you contribute to the world?
   - Have you considered any of the following?
     - Writing a book, newsletter, or article for publication
     - Setting up a trust fund for a friend or relative's child
     - Creating or contributing to a scholarship fund at a university or college
     - Helping to fund a public human service agency
     - Participating in a research project sponsored by a local college
     - Sponsoring a child overseas with small monthly contributions
     - Volunteering for a nonprofit organization

CELEBRATING CHILD-FREE LIVING

1. Depending on your infertility diagnosis, consider what forms of birth control you will use.

2. Inform your friends and your family members of your decision to become child-free.

3. Create a new identity through affirmation. For example: "I am a responsible, nurturing person, and my ability to nurture makes a difference in the world."

4. Congratulate yourself for transforming your loss into a gain.

5. Commemorate your decision through a special celebration, vacation, or both.

ADOPTION READINESS

We are sure your clients have heard both positive and negative things about adoption, and this conflicting information is confusing. The following questions are designed to help your clients understand what they can expect when parenting a child that is not biologically connected to them (although the child may be biologically connected to their partner). Remember, your clients must have a solid understanding and acceptance of who they are in order to help their adopted child develop a healthy self-concept. If the answers to the questions are primarily affirmative, your clients are likely to be an appropriate resource for an adopted child. If, however, the answers indicate that your clients perceive parenting as a duty and children as a liability and an obligation, your clients are not ready to consider this avenue to parenting. These clients should, in fact, look at the child-free living questionnaire to see if they wouldn't be more comfortable in a nontraditional parenting role.

Adoption Readiness Questionnaire

1. Does your lifestyle accommodate children?
2. Do you perceive parenting as the fulfillment of a dream (or as a duty)?
3. Do you view children as an asset (or a liability)?
4. If you are married, do you and your spouse share similar ideas about child rearing?
5. Do you have the time to devote to a child's ever-changing needs?
6. Do you feel that raising a child is a privilege (or an obligation)?
7. Do you feel comfortable parenting a child who is not born to you?
8. Are you able to fully embrace the background and heritage of your adopted child?
9. Are you adopting to solve problems or fill an empty life? The fuller your life is, the more you will be able to give your child.
10. Do you like who you are as the total of all of your experiences, *including* your experience with infertility?
11. Will you be able to talk openly and honestly with your child about adoption?
12. Will you be able to answer openly and honestly your child's questions about her birth parents?
13. Are you willing to facilitate your child's search for his birth parents when he reaches adulthood?
14. Will you be able to love this child unconditionally?
15. Does your partner want to adopt as much as you do?
16. Is your (marital) relationship stable enough to include a child?

ADOPTING A CHILD

This exercise is designed to inform your clients about the possible conditions that might be present in the child they are considering for adoption, or possible conditions in the child's family of origin. It is used in conjunction with the adoption readiness questionnaire as a reality check or "wake-up call" when clients are trying to decide if they can parent a child that is not biologically connected to them.

Adoption Worksheet

1. Please indicate which of the following you are willing to accept:

   Male   Twins

   Female   Sibling (indicate number of siblings)

   Caucasian   Hispanic

   Black   Asian

   Biracial   Multiracial

2. Age range: Minimum: Maximum:

3. In the following list, check the medical issues in the child that you are willing to consider:

   Low birth weight   Serious, correctable medical
                               condition
   Unknown medical
   prognosis   No prenatal care

   Minor, correctable   Noncorrectable birth defects
   medical condition
                               Emotional or psychological
   Special learning or   problems
   educational needs
                               HIV-positive or AIDS
   Hepatitis A, B, C

4. In the following list, check the circumstances of conception that you are willing to consider:

   Rape   Incest   Unknown paternity

5. In the following list, check the medical issues in birth parents that you are willing to consider. These factors may be present in one or both birth parents but do not necessarily affect the child.

Alcohol use during pregnancy	Alcohol use, not during pregnancy
Drug use during pregnancy	Drug use, not during pregnancy
Little or no information available on birth mother	Little or no information available on birth father
Mental illness	Sexually transmitted diseases
HIV-positive or AIDS	

6. Additional comments:

AFFIRMATIONS

Using daily affirmations can be an effective way for clients to begin altering the way they see themselves. They use new, positive language that empowers their behavior despite their experience with infertility. In a sense, affirmations rewrite the old, self-defeating script clients once used to define themselves. If clients use them regularly, affirmations become the natural way in which clients see themselves and their ability to effect change.

Affirmations

- It is OK to feel and express anger about the infertility.
- I have the right to take care of myself without feeling guilty or selfish.
- My self-worth does not depend on whether or not we (I) get pregnant.
- I lovingly take care of my body, my mind, and my emotions.
- I love and approve of myself.
- I will orchestrate my life and create balance from within.
- Today I open myself to new beliefs.
- I am capable of making changes in my life.
- I will decide which areas of my life I can control and which areas I cannot control.
- I will allow myself to experience the richness of my emotions.
- I claim my freedom from isolation.

- Today I am learning to flow with the current of life.
- I freely choose that which is best for me.
- My life is shaped by my choices, not by my predicaments.
- Today I affirm my right to make decisions.
- I give myself permission to be who I am.
- Today I take charge of my own life.
- It is safe for me to express my feelings appropriately.
- Today I have the courage to view life with realistic expectations.
- I am intelligent, courageous, and worthy, even if I do not become a parent.
- I feel free to move on to healthier ideas, thoughts, and emotions.
- Today I will listen attentively to all those I come in contact with.
- Today I will respect my body, my physical self.
- I make decisions confidently.
- I feel complete today, fulfilled and loved.
- I create my own happiness and do not rely on others to make me happy.
- I see the many things I can learn from others.
- I can make my dreams become reality.
- I possess the courage to choose the direction of my life.
- I have a clear, well-defined sense of myself.
- I feel good about myself today, and live with my pride.
- Today I let go of the things I cannot control.
- Wonderful choices are available to me.
- I am on a journey to discover the strong inner me.
- I have the strength and skill to deal with whatever comes my way.
- I rejoice in being a woman (man).
- I am willing to grow up and take responsibility for my life.
- I choose to live fully in the present.
- I am a worthy person, with or without a biological child.

USING BOOKS AND MOVIES

You can use books and movies in the same way that you use metaphors with your clients. You can assign specific titles to clients when you know they will receive a message that is difficult to convey in any other way. Clients usually perceive reading or viewing a movie as enjoyable homework that is neither threatening nor demanding. We have collected a repertoire of movies and fiction and nonfiction books that we refer to as nontraditional recommendations, because the subjects have nothing to do with infertility. We believe that it is easier for clients to experience the trials of characters whose predicament or message seems unrelated to theirs.

After clients have viewed the suggested film or read the book, you can discuss the story, characters, and main themes in therapy together. If your clients do not make the association between the story or themes and their own situation, you can facilitate that connection. The reading and viewing lists that appear in Appendix A are of titles that our clients have read and viewed. Of course, we have interpreted each film or book, and in no way does our use of the book or film constitute the "true meaning" of the creator. With this in mind, you will want to review these titles yourself as well as add others that you find appropriate for your clients who are experiencing infertility.

Here we provide one example of how we might use one of these titles with our clients. When we ask our clients to view *Mr. Holland's Opus,* it is usually at a point in therapy when clients have developed an objective look at their experience with infertility. This is because the story invites viewers to reframe their own experience with infertility, just as Mr. Holland has reframed his life experience.

Mr. Holland is a pianist with a vision. He dreams of living a life in which he can compose and perhaps make a major contribution to his field. But like many people, Mr. Holland is unable to work at the piano full-time, and takes a teaching job in order to pay the bills and support his growing family. He expects that in his spare time he will compose and develop his art. Unfortunately, the concept of spare time is an illusion, and Mr. Holland is unable to devote his life to composition. As Mr. Holland ages, and viewers witness the relationships he develops with his students, one senses that he is both satisfied with his work and frustrated by his inability to fully pursue his dream. When the music department is eliminated from the school where Mr. Holland teaches, he is forced to retire. In recognition of his contribution to the student body, all of his former students gather to perform Mr. Holland's opus in a farewell assembly.

The point the story appears to make is that dreams do not necessarily come true by the means we expect them to. By the end of the movie, Mr. Holland realizes that he did indeed make a profound impact in his chosen field and that his students were the opus he had always intended to create.

For clients who have dreamed of coming to parenting through biology, and receive an infertility diagnosis, it can be difficult to recognize that the dream of parenting can be achieved through other paths. We use the story of Mr. Holland's opus to illustrate the importance of remaining open. Otherwise, people risk taking their gifts for granted and overlooking the possibilities that surround them. For clients who are experiencing infertility, alternatives to biological parenting may elude them if they remain fixed on the path on which their dream was originally created. Watching the dawning of Mr. Holland's recognition that his dream did in fact come true can be empowering for clients who are able to make the connection that their dreams can come true, too, if they remain willing to explore all the possibilities available to them.

Suggested Viewing and Reading Lists

SUGGESTED VIEWING

How to Make an American Quilt. Uses a patchwork quilt as a metaphor for how lives are pieced together by random events that inevitably create a beautiful work.

Mr. Holland's Opus. Suggests that dreams come true in disguises and on different paths than those we expected.

Much Ado About Nothing. Profiles miscommunications and misperceptions (intentional and unintentional), and how they influence our choices and sometimes result in changing our reality.

Ordinary People. A portrayal of individual responses to the accidental death of a child.

Remains of the Day. Among other points, this film highlights the importance of self-expression and the consequences of culturally and self-imposed silence.

Shadowlands. Illustrates the risks and benefits of letting go of the fear of losing something you love.

Slingblade. Portrays trauma, isolation, and the power of acceptance of ourselves and others to change and shape us.

The Unbearable Lightness of Being. A glimpse into a world in which lives are shaped by irrevocable choices and events. (The title is best explained by author Milan Kundera on pp. 1–8 of the book on which the film is based.)

What's Eating Gilbert Grape? A tragic example of an individual who cannot get outside herself because of her physical limitations.

SUGGESTED NONFICTION

Alcoholics Anonymous: The Big Book (3rd ed.), Alcoholics Anonymous World Services.

Man's Search for Meaning, Viktor E. Frankl. A personal account of a concentration camp survivor and his belief that the last of the human freedoms is the ability to "choose one's attitude in a given state of circumstances."

Mars and Venus in the Bedroom, John Gray. A guide to lasting romance and passion.

Revolution from Within, Gloria Steinem. Essays on the development of self-esteem. Focuses on the importance of learning to meet our own needs instead of looking outside ourselves for fulfillment.

The Road Less Traveled: A New Psychology of Love, Traditional Values and Spiritual Growth, M. Scott Peck. An inspiring approach to wholeness.

The 7 Habits of Highly Effective People: Powerful Lessons in Personal Change, Stephen R. Covey. Challenges the quick-fix mentality of our culture and provides holistic, integrated principles for effective change.

Shrapnel in the Heart, Laura Palmer. The stories behind mementos left at the Vietnam Veterans Memorial. The custom of leaving mementos to honor the dead is a powerful representation of our need to express grief in a tangible way.

The Tao of Pooh, Benjamin Hoff. How to stay happy and calm under all circumstances.

Wouldn't Take Nothing for My Journey Now, Maya Angelou. A collection of one-page essays about the power of spirituality to move and shape your life.

SUGGESTED FICTION

Anagrams, Lorrie Moore. The power of imagination and humor to cope with losses and unfulfilled hopes.

Anywhere but Here, Mona Simpson. Explores a mother-daughter relationship through the eyes of the daughter. A compelling account of a
mother's inability to see her child as anything other than an extension of herself, and a daughter's struggle to be both herself and
loved by her mother.

Aquamarine, Carol Anshaw. Explores a life-defining event from three distinct perspectives. Each perspective assumes that the main character
made a different choice at her "moment of decision."

Bastard out of Carolina, Dorothy Allison. A book about child abuse. The
heroine is the victim, and her determination to survive is inspiring.

The Bean Trees, Barbara Kingsolver. The story of a young woman in search
of freedom. Ironically, she discovers "freedom" in the additional responsibilities of parenting an abused child.

The Beet Queen, Louise Erdrich. A forty-year saga that portrays the persis-
tence of relationships, the wonder of random events, and the unend-
ing mystery of the human condition. This is a story about survival.

The Book of Ruth, Jane Hamilton. A beautiful and disturbing story of survival and of the heroine's tenacious search for answers and effective
coping mechanisms.

The Color Purple, Alice Walker. The tragic and inspiring story of a young
woman's journey toward a life of her own.

Gift from the Sea, Anne Morrow Lindbergh. Demonstrates how patience
and being open to life's gifts can serve us in our attempts to gain
inner peace and a sense of wholeness.

High Tide in Tucson, Barbara Kingsolver. Twenty-five essays chronicling the
author's search for meaning and answers in an unscrupulous world.
She finds her answers in places you would least expect.

Illusions: The Adventures of a Reluctant Messiah, Richard Bach. A fictional
account on the nature of coincidence and the belief that all things
happen for a reason.

Maybe the Moon, Armistead Maupin. A book about being defined as outside of normal, from the perspective of the person being defined.

Seize the Day, Saul Bellow. An original perspective on the ability to grasp
the moment.

She's Come Undone, Wally Lamb. A story of emotional liberation.

Stones from the River, Ursula Hegi. A portrait of a woman who feels exceptionally different, and of her discovery that feeling different is something all humans share. It is also a book about courage and triumph
over circumstances out of our control.

FURTHER READING FOR THERAPISTS

The following is a recommended reading list for therapists. These books can provide you with a comprehensive, holistic understanding of your clients, their trials, and their healing journeys, thereby augmenting your work with clients experiencing infertility.

Bass, E., and Davis, L. (1994). *The Courage to Heal: A Guide for Women Survivors of Child Sexual Abuse.* New York: HarperCollins.

Bassoff, E. S. (1991). *Mothering Ourselves: Help and Healing for Adult Daughters.* New York: Plume.

Burns, D. D. (1980). *Feeling Good: The New Mood Therapy.* New York: Morrow.

Covey, S. R. (1989). *The 7 Habits of Highly Effective People: Powerful Lessons in Personal Change.* New York: Simon & Schuster.

Covington, S. (1991). *Awakening Your Sexuality: A Guide for Recovering Women and Their Partners.* New York: HarperCollins.

Dass, R., and Gorman, P. (1985). *How Can I Help? Stories and Reflections on Service.* New York: Knopf.

Fitzgerald, T. (1995). *Beyond Victimhood: Embrace the Future.* Minneapolis, Minn.: Fairview Press.

Fleming, A. T. (1994). *Motherhood Deferred: A Woman's Journey.* New York: Putnam.

James, J. W., and Cherry, F. (1988). *The Grief Recovery Handbook: A Step-by-Step Program for Moving Beyond Loss.* New York: HarperCollins.

Kottler, J. A. (1994). *Beyond Blame: A New Way of Resolving Conflicts in Relationships.* San Francisco: Jossey-Bass.

Mayeroff, M. (1971). *On Caring.* New York: HarperCollins.

Peck, M. S. (1978). *The Road Less Traveled: A New Psychology of Love, Traditional Values and Spiritual Growth.* New York: Simon & Schuster.

Rando, T. A. (1984). *Grief, Dying and Death: Clinical Interventions for Caregivers.* Champaign, Ill.: Research Press.

Rando, T. A. (1988). *How to Go on Living When Someone You Love Dies.* New York: Bantam Books.

Reynolds, M. (ed.). (1991). *Erotica: Women's Writings from Sappho to Margaret Atwood.* New York: Ballantine.

Satir, V. (1976). *Making Contact.* Berkeley, Calif.: Celestial Arts.

Shapiro, C. H. (1993). *When Part of the Self Is Lost: Helping Clients Heal After Sexual and Reproductive Losses.* San Francisco: Jossey-Bass.

Siegel, B. S. (1986). *Love, Medicine and Miracles: Lessons Learned About Self-Healing from a Surgeon's Experience with Exceptional Patients.* New York: HarperCollins.

Tatelbaum, J. (1980). *The Courage to Grieve: Creative Living, Recovery, and Growth Through Grief.* New York: HarperCollins.

Viorst, J. (1986). *Necessary Losses: The Loves, Illusions, Dependencies and Impossible Expectations That All of Us Have to Give Up in Order to Grow.* New York: Simon & Schuster.

Walsh, F., and McGoldrick, M. (Eds.). (1991). *Living Beyond Loss: Death in the Family.* New York: Norton.

Wolf, N. (1992). *The Beauty Myth.* New York: Doubleday.

Worden, J. W. (1991). *Grief Counseling and Grief Therapy: A Handbook for the Mental Health Practitioner.* New York: Springer.

SUGGESTED READING FOR THE USE OF METAPHORS IN TREATMENT

Barker, P. (1985). *Using Metaphors in Psychotherapy.* New York: Brunner/Mazel.

Cox, M., and Theilgaard, A. (1984). *Shakespeare as Prompter: The Amending Imagination and the Therapeutic Process.* Bristol, Pa.: Taylor & Francis.

Cox, M., and Theilgaard, A. (1987). *Mutative Metaphors in Psychotherapy: The Aeolian Mode.* New York: Routledge.

Gordon, D. (1978). *Therapeutic Metaphors.* Cupertino, Calif.: Meta.

Kelly, G. (1992). *The Psychology of Personal Constructs.* New York: Routledge.

Kopp, R. R. (1995). *Metaphor Therapy: Using Client-Generated Metaphors in Psychotherapy.* New York: Brunner/Mazel.

Resources

Adoptive Families of America (AFA)
3333 Highway 100 North
Minneapolis, MN 55422
Phone: 612–537–0316
An excellent resource for books, tapes, and adoption information packets. They publish an informative and practical bimonthly magazine for those touched by adoption. AFA also sponsors an annual national conference on adoption issues.

American Society for Reproductive Medicine
408 12th Street SW, Suite 203
Washington, DC 20024–2125
Phone: 202–863–2439
Fax: 202–484–4039
Web: www.asrm.com
An international organization of professionals who have an interest in family planning and reproductive health. Provides pamphlets on a range of topics in their Patient Information Series. The pamphlets are clearly written, educational, and extremely helpful for patients and

therapists alike. Pamphlets are available on the following topics: adoption, artificial insemination, birth defects of the female reproductive system, endometriosis, overview of infertility, coping and decision making after an infertility diagnosis, IVF and GIFT, menopause, miscarriage, ovulation detection and drugs, donor insemination, tubal factor infertility, and age and fertility.

The Childfree Network
7777 Sunrise Blvd., no. 1800
Citrus Heights, CA 95610
Phone: 916–773–7178
Provides a quarterly newsletter with articles on the beneficial and practical facets of life without children. Information is not necessarily specific to members who have experienced infertility.

The Compassionate Friends
National Office
P.O. Box 3696
Oakbrook, IL 60522
Phone: 708–990–0010
Web: www.compassionatefriends.org
An international self-help organization for parents who have experienced the death of a child. Some chapters have separate groups for siblings. Focuses on the trauma and grief that parents and siblings experience after the death of a child or sibling.

Ferre Institute
258 Genesee St., Suite 302
Utica, NY 13502
Phone: 315–724–4348
Web: members.aol.com/ferreinf/ferre.html
Provides education, information, and a newsletter on the psychological, social, and medical aspects of infertility and reproduction.

Infertility Network
160 Pickering St.
Toronto, Ont. M4E317 Canada
Phone: 416–691–3611
Fax: 416–690–8015
Provides support and information to people experiencing infertility. Develops public understanding and awareness of infertility as a medical

condition. Offers seminars, support groups, and a buddy system for members. Home page on the Web offers information and referral sources on both adoption and infertility.

National Council for Adoption
1930 17th Street NW
Washington, DC 20009
Phone: 202–328–1200
Web: www.ncfa-usa.org
An organization that promotes adoption as a positive alternative for building a family. The council is made up of member agencies (and refers potential adoptive parents to member agencies in their area) and individuals who are supportive of a conservative stance on openness in adoption.

North American Council on Adoptable Children (NACAC)
970 Raymond Avenue, no. 106
St. Paul, MN 55114–1149
Phone: 612–644–3036
Advocates for special needs adoption. They publish an informative and supportive newsletter (*Adoptalk*) and hold an annual conference focusing on special needs adoption. This organization is well regarded in the adoption community and has a wealth of resources to offer parents, professionals, and educators.

Organization of Parents Through Surrogacy
National Headquarters
P.O. Box 213
Wheeling, IL 60090
Phone: 847–394–4116
Fax: 847–394–4165
Web: www.opts.com
A national, nonprofit, all-volunteer organization whose purpose is providing mutual support, networking, and information on surrogate parenting.

Pregnancy and Infant Loss Center
1415 East Wayzata Blvd., no. 22
Wayzata, MN 55391
Provides information on reproductive losses that is appropriate for both families and therapists.

RESOLVE, Inc.
1310 Broadway
Somerville, MA 02144–1731
Helpline: 617–623–0744
Fax: 617–623–0252
Web: www.resolve.org
RESOLVE is a nationwide organization that provides information, referrals, support, and advocacy for people who are experiencing infertility. Their newsletter and fact sheets are available to the general public and can provide therapists with valuable information on new technology, educational workshops, and local resources.

vonEnde Communications
3211 St. Margaret Dr.
Golden Valley, MN 55422
Phone: 612–529–4493
Provides catalogs of audiotapes from various conferences and workshops on all aspects of infertility and adoption.

Alternatives to Biological Parenting
Practical Considerations

———

T his appendix provides you with information on the parenting options available through the latest reproductive technologies and adoption options.

REPRODUCTIVE TECHNOLOGIES

This section describes medical alternatives to biological parenting. The procedures discussed here are classified as *alternatives* to biological parenting because they require either donor sperm, donor eggs, or both. Clients usually consider donor programs after fertility treatments have failed to result in a pregnancy using the male client's sperm and the female client's egg, or when a medical condition, such as sterility in the male, makes the possibility of conceiving a biological child of both parents highly unlikely or nonexistent.

Clients may consider one or more of the following donor alternatives: donor intrauterine insemination, assisted reproductive technologies, embryo adoption, or surrogacy.

Donor Intrauterine Insemination (DIUI)

DIUI is used for couples in which the male partner is sterile. The procedure consists of inserting donor sperm directly into the female partner's uterus through a catheter placed in the cervix. A child conceived through this procedure is the biological child of the female partner and the male donor.

Assisted Reproductive Technologies (ART)

Currently there are three ART options available. In vitro fertilization (IVF) is a procedure in which fertilization of the egg and sperm takes place in a petri dish. (*In vitro* means "in glass.") The fertilized egg is then transferred to the woman's uterus. In gamete intrafallopian transfer (GIFT), an egg and sperm are transferred to the fallopian tube, where fertilization occurs. The fertilized egg then travels down the tube to the uterus, where it implants and grows. In zygote intrafallopian transfer (ZIFT), an egg fertilized in vitro is transferred to the fallopian tube. In all of these procedures, the egg or sperm (or both) can come from a donor, and the woman who carries the pregnancy may be either the female partner or a surrogate mother.

Surrogacy

In choosing surrogacy, a couple has four options:

1. The surrogate mother is inseminated with the male partner's sperm and carries her and the male partner's biological child to term.

2. The surrogate, through ZIFT or IVF, carries the couple's adopted embryo to term.

3. The surrogate is inseminated with the female partner's egg and donor sperm, and carries the female partner's and the male donor's biological child to term.

4. The surrogate is inseminated with the male and female partners' fertilized egg and then carries the couple's biological child to term. (This last alternative is sometimes referred to as using a "hostess" uterus or a gestational carrier.)

Embryo Adoption

This alternative provides clients with the opportunity to adopt a fertilized egg from donors. The fertilized egg is then transferred to the female partner's uterus or fallopian tube through ZIFT or IVF. The child who is born to the "adopting" couple is the biological child of the male and female donor. This option may also be used with a surrogate mother.

Practical Considerations

When clients decide to pursue medical alternatives to biological parenting, they must sift through an overwhelming amount of material: medical information, variances in state laws, and information about individual donor programs. At the same time, clients must comprehend the technical nature of much of this information. The following discussion classifies the various factors that clients must consider before selecting a donor alternative. We have also included a list of resources that can provide both you and your clients with additional information about the medical alternatives to biological parenting.

Making a fully informed decision about pursuing a donor alternative requires that clients examine the pragmatic side of choosing to parent through one of these medical alternatives. From a practical standpoint, couples need to weigh the costs, success rates, and legal implications of each procedure. They must also evaluate the services provided by each medical facility they consider, and each facility's reputation. With their physicians, clients should determine which donor procedures are most appropriate for them and then identify programs that can meet their medical needs. Clients can find information about donor programs on the Internet and in books and articles. Support groups, medical professionals, or other parents who have chosen the donor option can also be valuable sources of information.

Costs and success rates vary by procedure, number of attempts, and by the clinic or medical facility that performs the procedure. Clients should request information, in writing, about the costs and success rates of every program they are seriously considering. Clients should compare costs and success rates among programs and check each program's statistics against the results of independent research projects (which can be found in medical journals). Because each couple's medical condition can increase or decrease the chances of success, clients should consult a trusted physician about their own odds of success in relation to the program's overall success rate.

Clients should also request information about the legal aspects of each procedure they are considering. The applicable laws and legal requirements focus on such issues as adoption of a child born through the embryo adoption procedure, the legality of surrogacy in the client's state of residence, and the process of terminating the parental rights of the biological (or donor) parent. The program's staff should be able to discuss the state laws about the procedures they perform and refer the client to an attorney who is experienced in these matters. However, if a client resides in another state, the program may not be able to provide information about laws in the client's state of residence. In any event, clients should seek legal advice from an attorney in their own state of residence as well as an attorney in the program's state of operation before contracting with a donor program.

Clients must consider both the practical and emotional aspects of the legal risks of using donor alternatives. We have already mentioned some legal issues, but even if clients receive sound legal advice prior to selecting a donor program, they are still at risk for legal complications after they contract with a donor or surrogate. In the following discussion we use the term *surrogate* to mean both a traditional surrogate mother and donors of eggs or sperm.

The successful execution of a surrogacy contract is defined as fulfillment of the obligation of the surrogate parent to relinquish (physically, legally, or both) all rights that she may have to her biological child. An unsuccessful outcome of a surrogacy contract is therefore defined as a challenge by the surrogate (biological) parent to the agreement to relinquish her legal rights. Although surrogacy programs have experienced very high rates of success (some report success rates as high as 99 percent), the consequences for parents involved in a surrogacy contract that goes awry can be emotionally and financially devastating. We cannot overemphasize the complexity of the legal risks that potential parents take when they pursue surrogacy or embryo adoption. Because each arrangement between a surrogate and the potential parents is unique, the legal risks also vary from case to case.

Many of us are aware of nationally publicized cases in which a surrogate parent has petitioned the court to recognize her rights to parent a child born through a surrogacy procedure. Clients should review their surrogacy contract with an attorney and ask questions about the legal ramifications when a contract is broken by a surrogate (or by the clients themselves), and what their legal options for recourse would be. When potential parents do not have a biological connection to the child, and sometimes even when one of them does, they can find themselves in a situation in which they have no legal recourse if the surrogate decides not to relinquish her legal rights. They may also find themselves co-parenting their child with a surrogate against their will. Although these cases may be the exception, when they occur they can be devastating for all the parties involved, and the child can wind up in the middle of a legal battle in which there are no "winners."

ADOPTION OPTIONS

This section defines domestic, international, and special needs adoption. It also discusses practical considerations for each option and provides suggestions for how clients can access resources.

Domestic Adoption

We define domestic adoption as adoption in which the birth parents, the child, and the adoptive parents all reside in the same country, and the adoption is facilitated and finalized in the same country. Domestic adoptions may include traditional agency adoptions and private or independent adoptions. Agencies that facilitate adoptions have also combined various elements of traditional and private adoptions, which are referred to as nontraditional agency adoptions. Any of these adoptions may also be a special needs adoption or a transracial or transcultural adoption.

TRADITIONAL AGENCY ADOPTIONS.   These are adoptions that are wholly facilitated by either private and public adoption agencies. Birth parents and adoptive parents both receive services from agency workers (which may include counseling, living and medical expenses for birth parents, and a home study and post-placement supervision for adoptive parents). Making matches between birth parents, their child, and the prospective adoptive parents is the responsibility of the agency workers. Adoptive parents and birth parents have varying degrees of influence over the matching process. Ultimately, however, the legal custody of the child is transferred from the birth parents to the agency, and the final decision about a suitable adoptive family belongs to the agency staff, with the approval of the court of jurisdiction.

PRIVATE OR INDEPENDENT ADOPTIONS.   These are adoptions that are facilitated with the assistance of an attorney. Much variation exists in these adoptions, as adoptions are regulated by states, and the state law is sometimes subject to the interpretation of county courts. (This is also true for traditional and nontraditional agency adoptions.) Private adoptions can include all of the following methods:

- Prospective adoptive parents advertise for or identify prospective birth parents and retain an attorney to facilitate the adoption.

- Attorneys advertise, recruit, and make matches between prospective adoptive parents and birth parents.

- A relative of the prospective adoptive parents asks them to adopt his or her child.

- Birth parents or prospective adoptive parents contact agencies after having matched themselves, in order to gain access to such services as counseling, home studies and post-placement supervision, and temporary foster care.

In the case of the latter type of private adoption, usually the agency becomes involved because local laws require that a child-placing agency provide certain services to the parties involved. In private adoptions, the prospective adoptive parents' attorney often takes on some of the responsibilities that are normally assumed by personnel in a traditional agency adoption (such as facilitating the termination of the birth parents' parental rights). These adoptions sometimes take place several months after the adoptive parents have taken physical custody of the child.

NONTRADITIONAL AGENCY ADOPTIONS.   These adoptions combine elements of traditional agency and private adoptions. In some cases they include traditional agency adoption services, but the adoptive parents may identify the birth parents. Other cases use a matching process that includes developing and using profiles on birth parents and adoptive parents. Both parties review these profiles; the birth parents select an adoptive family, and the adoptive parents agree to the match. Nontraditional agency adoptions usually include high degrees of contact (both initial and ongoing) and extensive sharing of identifying information between birth parents and adoptive parents. Depending on the local laws, an attorney may also be involved in the adoption process.

PRACTICAL FACTORS.   Clients considering domestic adoption as an alternative to biological parenting need to consider the financial obligations, adoption laws, time frames, and degree of openness (or contact) between them and the birth parents.

Some financial assistance may be available even if the child does not have special needs. Domestic adoptions can range in cost from approximately $1,000 to $30,000 or more. Costs vary depending on—but are not limited to—agency fees (generally, public agencies limit their fees, but the parents are responsible for legal costs); the special needs of the child; the birth parents' medical coverage or lack of it; state laws that regulate the types of birth parent expenses that adoptive parents can assume responsibility for; and whether or not any fees are reimbursed if an adoption is disrupted.

Clients also need to weigh the legal risks involved in each type of domestic adoption they are considering, because disrupted adoptions have consequences for everyone involved. Adoptive parents may suffer the loss of a child they have been parenting and nurturing, and the child may suffer the loss of the adoptive parents with whom he has bonded. A disrupted adoption can become one more loss in a series of significant losses. Because laws vary by state and county, clients should contact an attorney who is experienced in adoptions, an adoption agency, or the juvenile court in their county for more information about local laws.

Time frames vary by type of adoption, but generally speaking, private and nontraditional agency adoptions are less time-consuming than traditional agency adoptions. However, clients can expect the overall time frame to be lengthened (usually by three to ten days depending on the state) when they are trying to adopt a child who is born in another state. This delay occurs because adoptive parents must have Interstate Compact (ICPC) approval before they can take their adopted child from her state of birth to the adoptive parents' state of residence. ICPC is an agreement developed between states to monitor and ensure that adoption regulations are being met in state-to-state adoptions and that the necessary requirements for finalizing an adoption have been met.

The time frames are generally shorter in nontraditional and private adoptions because the agency or the adoptive parents can recruit birth parents on a nationwide basis, whereas recruitment by traditional agencies is usually limited to the state in which they operate. In addition, adoptive parents are only recruiting birth parents for themselves, whereas agencies are recruiting birth parents for all of the potential parents with whom they have contracted. Clearly, well-informed and organized adoptive parents can be more assertive and effective advocates than can the staff of an adoption agency.

ACCESSING RESOURCES.   Clients can access the resources listed in Appendix B or can begin to investigate domestic adoption by contacting the adoption resources (agencies, attorneys, adoption consultants) listed in their local phone book. Clients may also want to join a local support group and access referrals from other potential parents or the group's referral list. They can also research adoption on the Internet and at their local library. Most clients report that the most helpful information comes from other potential or parenting adoptive parents and that they feel most comfortable using a resource that another potential adoptive parent has recommended.

International Adoption

Choosing international adoption as a parenting option means raising a child who was not born in the same country as the one in which the adoptive parents reside. Most of the countries that participate in placing children internationally are third world countries or nations in conflict. For third world countries, international adoption can help reduce the infant mortality rate that results from poverty; for nations in conflict, placing war orphans internationally can provide children with a chance for a stable life. Parents who adopt foreign-born children are usually from industrialized nations such as the United States, Australia, Canada, and Western European countries.

Depending on the interpretation of local laws and on the official who oversees each jurisdiction, international adoptions can be facilitated privately by attorneys, by public officials, and by licensed and nonlicensed child-placing agencies. Prospective adoptive parents usually choose a program (or professional) based on its ability to meet their specific needs for the particular child they wish to adopt.

ACCESSING RESOURCES.   Investigating international adoption often begins with a search through the yellow pages under "Adoption." Prospective parents will find listings for both attorneys and agencies. It has become increasingly common for adoption facilitators to participate in consumer hotlines: clients call one number and hear the numerous options available to them. Clients tell us that these services can be overwhelming and confusing and that they usually need to have a consultant untangle the yards of information received.

Adoption consultants are also listed under "Adoption" in the phone book. They may also be cross-referenced under "Counseling," "Consulting," or "Marriage and Family Counseling." Consultants can provide direction and focus for overwhelmed clients. In our practice, we make direct referrals to a pool of resources that we feel certain can help clients narrow the field of possibilities. These referrals always include adoption publications that list international child-placing agencies throughout the nation, clients who have already adopted internationally, and local community adoption-support groups.

Our clients tell us that nothing is more helpful than talking to people who have already done what they hope to do. Only veteran adoptive parents can provide the details that clients considering international adoption really need in order to transform theories and dreams into facts and realities. In addition, clients who have experienced infertility and wonder if they will ever experience parenting are most encouraged by seeing other successful adoptions.

WEIGHING PRACTICAL FACTORS.   We are fond of referring to international adoption as the closest thing clients are going to get to a guarantee of parenting. We say this because there are so many programs placing so many children worldwide that there seems to be a program for everyone. Although every child-placing agency and every country has specific requirements that clients must meet regarding marital status, age, years married, or age difference between prospective parents and child, there is a broad range of acceptable variables.

In addition to considering program requirements, clients must also consider the costs associated with an international adoption. Although costs vary, legal, agency, foreign source, document preparation, and travel fees usually average between $15,000 and $25,000 for the adoption of a relatively healthy, young child. The federal government and many states have tax reimbursement programs for adoption-related expenses. Also, some employers reimburse portions of their employees' adoption costs. Whether or not clients are able to receive tax credits or reimbursements, however, they must be prepared to incur all expenses at the outset of the adoption process.

Although it can be costly, adopting internationally doesn't usually present the same time constraints that domestic adoption programs can. The number of available foreign-born children far surpasses the number of parents waiting to adopt. Unlike a domestic program where clients may wait for years, clients who choose to adopt internationally *usually* do not wait more than one year from the time they are approved as an adoptive resource and their documents completed. The actual time spent in the process, of course, will vary from one program and country to another.

Another factor that can influence the time clients spend waiting is unforeseen changes in the laws of the foreign country. Foreign officials evaluate their adoption procedures on an ongoing basis. Occasionally, clients get caught in the middle of changing laws. In the best situations, adoptions already in process are allowed to finalize under the former law. In the worst situations, programs close and clients lose the children they were assigned to.

Besides the time spent preparing and waiting to adopt, clients must also consider the time and expense involved in traveling to another country to participate in the legal process. Some countries require one trip; the adoption may take as few as three days to complete the process, but others may take as long as three to four weeks. Other countries may require two appearances from adopting parents. In these situations, the transfer of custody takes place during the first trip. The child is then placed in foster care, and the adopting parents return home. Ten days to three months later, parents travel again to finalize the adoption. Some countries allow an agency representative to escort the child to the adoptive parents' country of origin, thereby eliminating the need for travel by the adopting parents. In these cases, although clients will not incur the expense of their own travel, they are expected to assume the costs of having their child brought home.

Although most international adoptions are finalized in the foreign country prior to the child's exit from her birth nation, we recommend that adoptive parents have their adoptions recognized in their local courts. If the foreign adoption process is in compliance with the adoption laws of the state the parents live in, parents can file a one-count petition in the local court to have the adoption recognized. If the foreign process is not in compliance with state laws, clients should file a two-count petition that (1) transfers custody to the adopting parents and (2) finalizes the adoption. This latter process is called a readoption. Whether recognizing the foreign adoption in the local court or readopting, both processes give the adopted child all of the same rights that other citizens in that state have. These rights usually include voting rights, amended birth certificates, and uncontestable inheritance rights. In order to receive national citizenship, the adopted child must be naturalized through their country's immigration and naturalization services department.

Special Needs Adoption

Special needs is a term used to describe children who are hard to place for adoption. These children may have medical, emotional, and social problems; may be members of a minority race or culture; may be part of a sibling set; or are older than one year of age. They are considered hard to place because they do not fit the description of a "healthy Caucasian infant." Caucasian couples experiencing infertility are more likely to pursue infertility treatment than couples of other ethnic backgrounds. When treatment is unsuccessful, most Caucasian couples try to adopt a healthy Caucasian infant in order to create the experience of traditional parenting that most closely emulates the family the couple would have had. The demand for healthy Caucasian infants is therefore higher than the demand for children with special needs.

Few adoptive resources are available for children with special needs. One reason permanent homes are hard to find is that the child's special needs often require an enormous financial commitment from parents. Financial support from both federal and state programs is available, however, so that no child with special needs is ineligible for adoption solely on the basis of financial concerns. Thus, clients who doubt their financial ability to parent a child who needs extensive medical, psychological, or institutional care can in reality usually do so.

Another reason permanent homes are hard to find is that the long-term prognosis for the child with special needs is often unknown. Many prospective adoptive parents are admittedly unable to commit to a child with a guarded prognosis. And of course, all children with special needs require flexible and committed parents who feel able to accept any outcome of their adopted child's special situation. This flexibility and level of commitment often develops through education.

WEIGHING PRACTICAL FACTORS.   The *process* of adopting a child with special needs (as opposed to the *raising* of a child with special needs) does not usually create an enormous financial burden for prospective parents. Most public and private agencies placing domestic-born special needs children receive private, corporate, or government subsidies (or some combination of subsidies) that reimburse them for the expenses of foster care and parent education. Thus, agencies do not have to pass these expenses on to their adoptive clients. Foreign-born children who have moderate to severe medical problems, who are part of a sibling group, or who are over eight years of age are often placed without the usual foreign-source and child-placing-agency fees. These fees are waived because the primary commitment of the agency and the child's country of origin is to having the child's special needs met. Many appropriate prospective adoptive families are discouraged by the fees they expect to pay when pursuing adoption. However, most special needs adoption programs eliminate this concern.

Another factor to consider with special needs adoption programs is that although there are always children in need of permanent homes, clients' waiting time for an assignment to a child will vary. Clients considering adopting domestic-born children with special needs may wait longer than they expect to. Contrary to what many clients believe, there is no "list" on which clients waiting to adopt are placed. If there were a list, clients would, at the very least, expect to move up on the list. Instead, after clients have completed the home study process, they are added to a *pool* of other waiting parents. Clients are prospectively matched with various children according to their responses on the adoption worksheet (discussed in Chapter Seven and provided in Chapter 11). All of the adoption professionals involved review the factors that waiting parents are willing to consider, along with the special needs the child presents. Thus, the time that clients spend waiting to be matched with a domestic-born child can seem long because the task of determining the best possible placement for a child is arduous and time-consuming. After waiting parents are matched with a child, the process of pre-placement visits begins.

Pre-placement visits are designed to help prospective parents and their prospective child get to know one another. This process is especially important for children who have a history of living in numerous homes or who have endured abuse and/or neglect. These children have experienced very little to assure them that the prospective adopting parents can be trusted to provide a safe and stable home. Depending on the comfort level of everyone involved, pre-placement visits with domestic-born children can take place over weeks or months. When clients thoroughly understand the purpose of pre-placement visits, their anxiety to have the child placed in their home immediately is usually assuaged.

After children are placed in their adoptive homes, post-placement visits and supervision ensue. These visits are designed to support each family member in his or her adjustment to the adoptive placement. Although laws vary, most agencies that facilitate domestic special needs adoptions require that at least one year pass after the child has been placed before recommending to the local court that the adoption be finalized. The year-long time frame is not chosen arbitrarily. One complete cycle of anniversaries both of traumatic events and of celebrations must pass before family members can begin to understand one another. We encourage our clients to use post-placement supervision as a source of support, resources, and guidance.

ACCESSING RESOURCES.   Clients usually learn about special needs adoption from their friends or from social workers. Although clients seldom initially consider this type of adoption, information and education often have a positive impact on clients' willingness to consider parenting a child with special needs as a viable alternative to biological parenting.

Extraordinary recruitment measures are often used in order to secure an adoptive family for domestic-born children with special needs. Children might be featured on television or included in a statewide registry that usually includes medical, psychosocial, and developmental information as well as the children's photograph. Some clients are drawn to specific children through these television spots and registries and will initiate the adoption process for a particular child.

For our clients considering special needs adoption, we provide referrals that include adoption publications and lists of public and private child-placing agencies throughout the state and the country. We also facilitate contact between prospective parents and clients who have already adopted children with special needs. In addition, we recommend participation in local community adoption-support groups for parents of children with special needs.

⟿ References

Allison, D. (1993). *Bastard out of Carolina.* New York: Penguin, p. 213.

American Psychiatric Association. (1994). *Diagnostic and Statistical Manual of Mental Disorders* (4th ed.). Washington, D.C.: American Psychiatric Association.

American Society for Reproductive Medicine. (1996). *Age and Fertility: A Guide for Patients.* Birmingham, Ala.: American Society for Reproductive Medicine.

Bon Breathnach, S. (1995). *Simple Abundance.* New York: Warner Books.

Conrad, J. (1911). *Heart of Darkness.* New York: MacMillan.

Frankl, V. (1959). *Man's Search for Meaning: An Introduction to Logotherapy.* Boston: Beacon Press.

Herman, J. L. (1992). *Trauma and Recovery: The Aftermath of Violence: From Domestic Abuse to Political Terror.* New York: Basic Books.

Lindbergh, A. M. (1991). *Gift from the Sea.* New York: Vintage, pp.16–17.

Nietzsche, F. (1899). *Twilight of the Idols.* Edinburgh: W. Blackwood and Sons.

Offit, A. K. (1981). *Night Thoughts: Reflections of a Sex Therapist.* New York: Congdon & Lattes.

Osbon, D. K. (Ed.). (1992). *Reflections on the Art of Living: A Joseph Campbell Companion.* New York: HarperCollins.

Steinem, G. (1992). *Revolution from Within: A Book of Self-Esteem.* Boston: Little, Brown.

Suzuki, S. (1970). *Zen Mind, Beginner's Mind.* New York and Tokyo: Weatherhill.

Webster's New World Dictionary of American English, Third College Edition. (1988). New York: Simon & Schuster.

Williamson, M. (1992). *A Course in Miracles: A Return to Love.* New York: HarperCollins.

⌁ About the Authors

Lara L. Deveraux received her B.A. in social work from Idaho State University and her M.S.W. degree from George Warren Brown School of Social Work at Washington University in St. Louis.

Ann Jackoway Hammerman received her B.S. degree from the University of Kansas and her M.S.W. from the George Warren Brown School of Social Work at Washington University in St. Louis, Missouri.

In March 1994, Hammerman and Deveraux opened a private counseling practice in order to provide pragmatic support to people with fertility problems. In addition, they became a licensed child-placing facility in February 1995 to provide clients with a comprehensive source for all services relative to parenting. They have been collecting ideas and collaborating on this professional manual for nearly a decade and are considered two of the community's experts on infertility and adoption issues. In addition to regular speaking engagements at the local chapter of RESOLVE, International Families (a community support group), and child-placing agencies throughout the country, Deveraux and Hammerman fulfill all administrative and marketing responsibilities for their growing clinical practice.

──ᴘ── Index

Donation alternatives. *See* Egg and
sperm donation
Donor intrauterine insemination
(DIUI), 293. *See also* Alternatives
to biological parenting; Egg and
sperm donation; Reproductive
technologies
Donor relationships, 166–169, 295–296.
See also Surrogates
Donor sperm, 151

E

Education. *See* Information gathering;
Resources; Self advocacy; Sex
education
Educational experience, in autobiography, 263
Egg and sperm donation, 151–152,
292–296; costs of, 294–295; decision
making for, 165–169; emotional
considerations in, 165–169; grief
over loss of potential biological
child and, 166; information gathering and self-advocacy for, 240–245,
294; practical considerations in,
165, 292, 294–296; relationship issues in, 166–169; success rates of,
294–295; telling child about, 167–
168. *See also* Alternatives to biological parenting; Reproductive technologies; Surrogacy; Surrogates
Egg freezing, 118, 151
Embryo adoption, 294
Emotional detachment, 1–2
Emotional expression: in grief process,
113, 114, 126; in infertility counseling, 14–15; of jealousy, 86–87; of
men, 76–77; of women, 68, 70,
77–78; writing assignments for,
17–18
Emotional expressiveness: of men,
76–77; of women, 68, 70, 77–78
Emotions, understanding the source of,
105. *See also* Anger
Empathy: demonstrating, 34–35; in
grief therapy, 119; versus projection,
34–35; versus sympathy, 35

Employment, and child-free living, 160
Empowerment: for effective self-
advocacy, 169–171; fostering, 19–25;
for integration of identity, 204–205;
nonendorsement and, 52–53; reframing for, 41–42. *See also* Responsibility; Self-advocacy
Endorsement/nonendorsement, 52–53
Erdrich, L., 285
Exercises, 257–282; for coping with
child's pregnancy, 198; for dealing
with insensitivity, 188; for decision
making, 49–50, 152–153; for decision making about adoption, 163,
224–227; for decision making
about child-free living, 158–159;
for decision making about medical
treatment, 152–154, 156–157; for
experiencing healthy sexuality, 140–
143, 148; for grieving at menopause,
177; for grieving reproductive loss,
109–110, 219, 223; for recurring
grief at anticipated life events, 176,
177; for recurring grief at unanticipated life events, 180–181, 185; use
of, 17–18. *See also* Adoption readiness questionnaire; Adoption worksheet; Affirmations; Autobiography;
Considering child-free living; Couples inventory; Decision-making
skills inventory; Financial assessment and planning form; Homework assignments; Integrity wheel;
Journal writing; Personal loss inventory; When to discontinue treatment
Experts, clients as, 13–14, 27

F

Families, blended, 26, 228, 229
Family, clients': in autobiography,
262–263; holidays with, 84–85; journal writing about, 260–261; managing questions from, 81–84
Family, culture's definition of, 158. *See
also* Couple relationship
Family discord/dysfunction: in child-
focused marriages, 73–74; infertility

118–121; for recurring grief, 176;
for reproductive loss, 109–127,
166; for specific reproductive
losses, 115–127; stages of grief
and, 110–114. *See also* Recurring
grief
Guiding skills, 40–53; of finding an appropriate context, 44–45; of finding
a manageable perspective, 43–44; of
metaphors and analogies, 45–47; of
pragmatic problem solving, 48–50;
of providing resources, 50–53, 169–
171; of reframing, 40–43. *See also*
Decision making; Problem solving;
Reframing; Skills, therapeutic
Guilt feelings: about abortion history,
88–89, 230–233; about birth control
history, 113; about post-conception
losses, 125; about sexual history,
87–90, 113

H

Hamilton, J., 285
Heart of Darkness (Conrad), 211
Hegi, U., 285
Heracleitus, 172
Herman, J. L., 95, 99
High Tide in Tucson (Kingsolver), 285
History, client: in assessment session,
212–217; infertility, 212–213; psy-
chosocial, 135–136, 143–144; rela-
tionship, 213; sexual, 87–90, 113;
of sexual abuse/assault, 26. *See also*
Couples inventory; Personal loss
inventory
Hobbies, in autobiography, 264
Hoff, B., 284
Holidays, 84–85
Homework assignments, 257–258; for
combined-diagnosis couples, 79–80;
for couple communication, 69–70;
for self-education about medical
treatment, 142. *See also* Autobiography; Exercises; Journal writing
How to Make an American Quilt, 283
Hysterectomy, 118, 119–120

I

Identity, 2, 3; accepting change and,
205–206; finding a context for, 45,
120; gender, 63–68; gender roles
and, 131–132, 137–140, 143,
235–236; grieving and, 204; infertility as a condition and, 12–16,
202–203; integrating infertility into,
12–13, 16, 114, 140–141, 202–207,
233–239; journal writing about,
261; regaining healthy, 202–207; role
of gender in formation of, 63–64;
sexual history integration in, 87–90;
sexuality integration in, 140–141,
143; tools for integration of, 18
Identity and infertility session, 233–
239; case study of, 234–239; exploring options in, 236–238; focus of,
234–236; purpose of, 233; task assignment in, 238
*Illusions: The Adventures of a Reluctant
Messiah* (Bach), 285
Impotency, in case study, 137–138, 237
In vitro fertilization (IVF), 151, 293,
294; in self-advocacy case study,
240–245. *See also* Alternatives to
biological parenting; Egg and sperm
donation; Reproductive technologies
Infertility: accepting limitations of,
106–108; as condition versus definition of self, 12–16, 202–203, 233;
dilemmas of, 80–91; emotional reactions to, 1–2, 14–15; impact of,
on clients, 57–74, 102–109; as life
crisis, 91–95; marriage based on,
72–73, 114–115; primary, 116–117;
secondary, 117–118; sexual history
and, 87–90; sexuality and, 128–149;
specific responses to, 75–95; themes
of, 6–7. *See also* Identity; Loss; Reproductive loss
Infertility counseling: assessment
session of, 212–217; communication skills for, 32–40; for decision
making, 150–169, 223–228; guiding skills for, 40–53; for identity

integration, 202–207; for recurring grief, 172–201, 217–223; for reproductive loss and grief, 99–127, 217–223; session plans for, 211–256; for sexual relationships, 132–149; supportive, 31–32, 117–118; termination of, 250–256; therapist skills for, 31–53. *See also* Communication skills; Decision making; Grief therapy; Guiding skills; Identity; Infertility treatment; Recurring loss; Sexuality; Skills; Session plans; Therapeutic relationship

Infertility history-taking, 212–213

Infertility Network, 289–290

Infertility treatment: client empowerment in, 19–25; client as expert in, 13–14, 27; dealing with loss in, 16–19; exercises in, 17–18, 257–258; infertility as a condition and, 12–16; model of, 4–5, 11–30; promoting acceptance in, 14–16, 20–21; promoting responsibility-taking in, 21–24, 204–205; self-advocacy and, 25; special concerns and, 26–30, 228–233; themes of, 6, 11–12; tools of, 6, 18; traditional models of, 1–3. *See also* Exercises; Infertility counseling; Medical treatment

Information, 25; brokering, 169–170; client assertiveness for obtaining, 170–171. *See also* Resources

Injustice, 90–91, 111

Insensitivity of other people, 185–189; towards child-free couples, 185–187; towards clients who are parents, 187–189. *See also* Family, client's; Friends; Questions

Integrity wheel, 79–80, 269–271; and autobiography, 261; for couple partnership, 238; examples of use of, 235, 238; for grief at divorce, 184–185; for grief at menopause, 177; for grief at retirement, 177; for integration of sexuality, 140–141; sample, 270

Intense emotion, 1–2

International adoption, 162–163, 299–302; accessing resources about, 299–300; finances of, 300; legal issues of, 301–302; practical considerations of, 300–302; time frames of, 300–301

Interpretation, and reflective listening, 37

Interstate Compact (ICPC) approval, 298

Intimacy: impact of infertility on, 132–133; reclaiming, 141. *See also* Couple relationship; Sexuality

Isolation, 58; and dealing with family-focused holidays and celebrations, 84–85, 103–106; dealing with feelings of, 105–106; reproductive loss and, 103–106

J

"Jan and David" case study, 48–50, 224–228

Jealousy, 86–87, 111

Journal articles, 51

Journal writing, 258–261; assigned at assessment session, 216, 217; about coping mechanisms, 259–260; for dealing with insensitivity of others, 188; examples of use of, 216, 217, 231, 244; about family, 260–261; for grief at child's pregnancy, 198; for grief at death of a loved one, 176; for grief at divorce, 184; for grief at menopause, 177; for grieving post-conception losses, 126–127; guidelines for, 258–261; for marriage based on infertility, 72–73; post-termination, 253; questions to address in, 259–261; reflections in, 261; about self-esteem, 259; for special concerns, 231

K

"Kae and Don" case study, 195–198, 217–223

Kingsolver, B., 285

Kübler-Ross, E., 110

81–84; right to, 81; and sexuality, 133–134, 141–142
Proactivity, 204–205. *See also* Empowerment
Problem solving, pragmatic, 48–50, 152–153, 224, 227. *See also* Decision making
Professional boundaries, 27–30
Projection, therapist, 34–35, 42. *See also* Countertransference
Psychological instability, 61–62
Psychosocial history, 135–136, 143–144
Psychosocial symptoms, 2–3

Q

Questions from family and friends: appropriate/inappropriate, 81; managing, 81–84, 188–189; prepared answers for, 83–84, 106; right to privacy and, 81; as triggers of recurring grief, 185–189

R

Rachel and Dean. *See* "Dean and Rachel"
"Rebecca" case study, 88–89, 230–233
Recognition, 20. *See also* Acceptance
Recurring grief: with adopted children, 165, 191–198; at anniversaries of previous losses, 174; at announcement of new reproductive technologies, 178–181; at anticipated life events, 173–177; with child-free living, 160, 191–198; coping with, 172–201; at death of a loved one, 174–176; at divorce, 183–185; due to changes in sexual functioning, 189–191; due to fertility of others, 198–201; due to insensitivity of others, 185–189; due to life events, 173–185; due to parenting stages, 191; versus initial grief, 172–173; at menopause, 176–177; at pregnancy of client's children, 165, 195–198, 217–223; at retirement, 177; session plan for, 217–223; at sexual activity of client's children, 165, 195–198;

triggers of, 173–201; at unanticipated life events, 178–185; at unexpected/unplanned pregnancy, 181–183. *See also* Grief; Loss; Reproductive loss
Referrals, 250; brokering information and, 169–170; making specific, 52–53. *See also* Organizations; Resources; Support groups
Reflective listening, 35–37; in grief therapy
Reframing, 40–43; cautions for, 42–43; for client empowerment, 41–42; in grief therapy, 119
Relationship history-taking, 212. *See also* Couples inventory
Relaxation techniques, 232
Religious views, in autobiography, 264
Reproduction, cultural attitudes about, 100–102
Reproductive loss: coping with, 99–127; cultural attitudes and, 100–102, 105, 106; defined, 99–100; deprivation and, 108–109; grieving process for, 109–114; impact of, on feminine identity, 66–67; impact of, on masculine identity, 65; impact of, recognizing, 102–109; intangible, 118–121; isolation and, 103–106; of loss of potential biological child, 115–127, 166; post-conception, 116, 121–127; pre-conception, 116–121; types of, 99–100; types of, working with specific, 115–127. *See also* Grief; Grief stagnation; Grief therapy; Loss; Recurring grief
Reproductive technologies, 151, 292–296; announcement of new, recurring grief at, 178–181; assisted, 293; decision making for, 165–169; and hysterectomy, 118; practical considerations of, 292, 294–296; self-advocacy and, 240–245; types of, 151, 293–294. *See also* Alternatives to biological parenting; Egg and sperm donation; Medical treatment; Surrogacy

Resentment, 111–112

Resolution, 1–2, 6; advocating acceptance over, 20–21, 202, 204

RESOLVE, Inc., 52, 216, 250, 252, 255, 291

Resources, 283–291; for adoption, 227, 299–300, 304; for alternatives to biological parenting, 53, 169–171; developing a catalogue of, 50–52; for donor programs, 294; general types of, 51; lists of, 283–291; for menopause support, 176–177; organizational, listed, 288–291; providing relevant, 50–53; referrals and, 52–53; for self-advocacy, 25, 169–170. *See also* Books; Movies; Organizations; Self-advocacy; Support groups

Responsibility, versus control, 21–24, 204–205, 219, 221–223. *See also* Empowerment

Retirement, as trigger of recurring grief, 177

Revolution from Within (Steinem), 128, 284

Rituals: for anniversaries of previous losses, 174; for dealing with loss, 18–19

Road Less Travelled, The (Peck), 284

S

Scars, from surgical procedures, 155–156

School, as trigger of recurring grief, 193–194

Secondary infertility, 117–118; acknowledging losses of, 120–121

Seize the Day (Bellow), 285

Self-actualization, 19

Self-advocacy, 25, 150, 239–240; for alternatives to biological parenting, 169–171, 239–240; skills for, 241. *See also* Empowerment; Resources

Self-advocacy session, 239–245; case study of, 240–245; exploring options in, 244; focus of, 241–244; purpose of, 240–245; task assignment in, 244–245

Self-definition, infertility as condition versus, 12–16, 202–203, 233. *See also* Identity

Self-disclosure, therapist, 28–29

Self-esteem, 128, 148–149, 259

Self-talk, therapist, 38

Session plans, 211–259; alternatives to biological parenting, 250–256; assessment, 212–217; decision-making, 223–228; financial planning, 245–250; follow-up, 253–256; grief, 217–223; infertility and identity, 233–239; self-advocacy, 239–245; special concerns, 228–233; termination, 250–256

7 Habits of Highly Effective People, The (Covey), 284

Sex education: of adopted children, 191, 194–195; ideal, 128–129

Sexual assault/abuse history, 26, 228, 230–233

Sexual function/dysfunction, 129; in case study, 137–138, 237; changes in, as trigger of recurring grief, 189–191

Sexual history, 87–90, 113, 230–233

Sexuality: barriers to healthy, 130–132; context of, 129, 130; counseling for, 135–149; creating boundaries between infertility and, 142–143; curiosity and, 130–131; ideal healthy, 128–129; impact of infertility on, 132–135, 136–140, 144–148; integration of, into whole identity, 140–141, 143; intimacy and, 132–133, 141; loss of privacy and, 58–59, 133–134, 141–142; maintaining privacy and, 141; medical treatment impact on, 58–59, 133–134, 142–143; pressure to conceive and, 134–134, 142–143; procreative roles and, 131–132, 137–140, 143; power struggles and, 145–148; psychosocial history-taking for, 135–136, 143–144; societal influences on, 130–131; tools for experiencing healthy, 140–143, 148. *See also* Couple relationship